Anatomy Cardiovascular System Label Practice

By K.R. Lefkowitz

Copyright © 2016 K.R. Lefkowitz

All rights reserved.
ISBN: 10: 1532985142
ISBN-13: 978-1532985140

CARDIOVASCULAR SYSTEM

1. AORTA & INTERCOSTAL
2. ARM - VENOUS DRAINAGE
3. ARTERIAL ANATOMY
4. ARTERIAL ANATOMY
5. ARTERIAL CIRCLE OF WILLIS
6. ARTERIAL CIRCLE OF WILLIS
7. ARTERIES - AB VISCERA
8. ARTERIES - BRAIN
9. ARTERIES - CIRCLE OF WILLIS
10. ARTERIES - CRANIAL
11. ARTERIES - EXT HEAD & NECK
12. ARTERIES - HEAD & NECK
13. ARTERIES - MAJOR
14. ARTERIES - NECK
15. ARTERIES - PALM & HAND
16. ARTERIES - ULNAR & RADIAL
17. ARTERY, VEIN & CAPILLARY
18. ATRIOVENTRICULAR NODE
19. AXILLARY ARTERY & VEIN
20. BLOOD CELLS
21. BLOOD VESSELS ANATOMY
22. BRACHIAL ARTERY
23. CARDIA MUSCLE HISTOLOGY
24. CARDIAC MUSCLE
25. CARDIOPULMONARY SYSTEM 1
26. CARDIOPULMONARY SYSTEM 2
27. CARDIOVASCULAR SYSTEM
28. CELIAC ARTERY
29. CONDUCTION SYSTEM 1
30. CONDUCTION SYSTEM 2
31. CORONARY ARTERIAL SYSTEM
32. CRANIAL CAVITY BASE
33. DEVELOPMENT OF FETAL HEART
34. ECHO-CARDIO - PARASTERNAL
35. ECHO-CARDIO - PLANES
36. EKG CURVES
37. FEAL CIRCULATION
38. HEAD - FALX CEREBRI
39. HEART - ANTERIOR WALL
40. HEART - CHAMBERS & VESSELS
41. HEART - DIAPHRAGM SURFACE 1
42. HEART DIAPHRAGM SURFACE 2
43. HEART - GREAT VESSELS
44. HEART - GREAT VESSELS
45. HEART - GREAT VESSELS
46. HEART - LEFT LATERAL
47. HEART - MUSCULATURE
48. HEART - POSTERIOR WALL
49. HEART - SECTION
50. HEART - STERNOCOSTAL
51. HEART & PRINCIPLE ARTERIES
52. HEART
53. HEART
54. HEART
55. HEART
56. HEART BLOOD FLOW
57. HEART CHAMBERS
58. HEART VALVES
59. HEPATIC PORTAL SYSTEM
60. LYMPHATIC SYSTEM OVERVIEW
61. LYMPHATICS - ABDOMINAL
62. RADIOGRAM - ANTEROPOSTERIOR
63. RADIOGRAM - L ANT OBLIQUE
64. RADIOGRAM R ANT OBLIQUE
65. SPLEEN
66. THORACIC BONES & HEART 1
67. THORACIC BONES & HEART 2
68. THORACIC BONES & HEART 3
69. THORACIC BONES & HEART 4
70. THORACIC CAGE
71. THORACIC PLANES
72. THORAX - CROSS SECTION
73. TORSO OF HEART 1
74. TORSO OF HEART 2

75. TORSO OF HEART 3
76. TORSO OF HEART 4
77. TORSO OF HEART 5
78. TORSO WITH RIBS & HEART 1
79. TORSO WITH RIBS & HEART 2
80. TORSO WITH RIBS & HEART 3
81. TORSO WITH RIBS & HEART 4
82. ULTRASOUND
83. VASCULATURE - ABDOMEN 1
84. VASCULATURE 0 ABDOMEN 2
85. VASCULATURE - KIDNEYS
86. VASCULATURE - THORAX
87. VASUCULTURE - THYROID GLAND
88. VEIN ANATOMY
89. VEIN ANATOMY 2
90. VENOUS DRAINAGE OF BRAIN
91. VENTRICLES

How To Use….

This book is mean't to be used for you to label and practice the components of the cardiovascular system. In going through your anatomy class and later in medical field you will need to know how to label the components, pictures of each system and know it inside and out. The best way is for you to label all the components that you know yourself and research the areas that you don't. Can you label all parts of the heart, ventricles, parties, veins, etc…? Can you recognize a picture and know immediately what it is? You can find the corresponding picture in the table of contents. Nothing is labeled on purpose. This is for you to label. For you to know. And what you don't know for you to research in your texts and find the answers. Through this way of learning and researching the parts you don't know, allows you to actually learn it and have it stored in long term memory. This active way of learning will in the long term be beneficial beyond belief in your future career or knowledge. Mark the pages, make notes, and use this practice book and pictures to help you understand the parts of the anatomy.

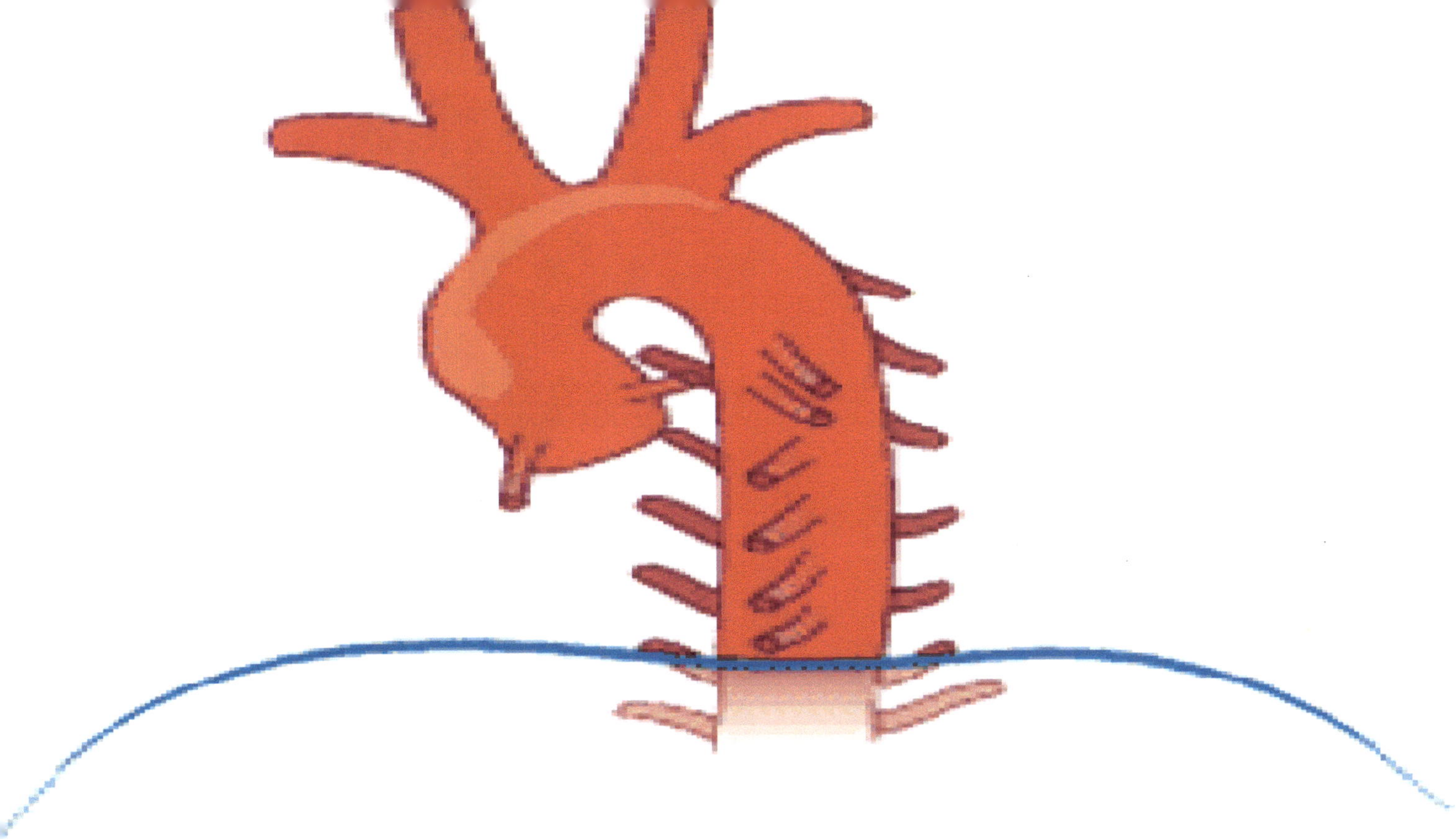

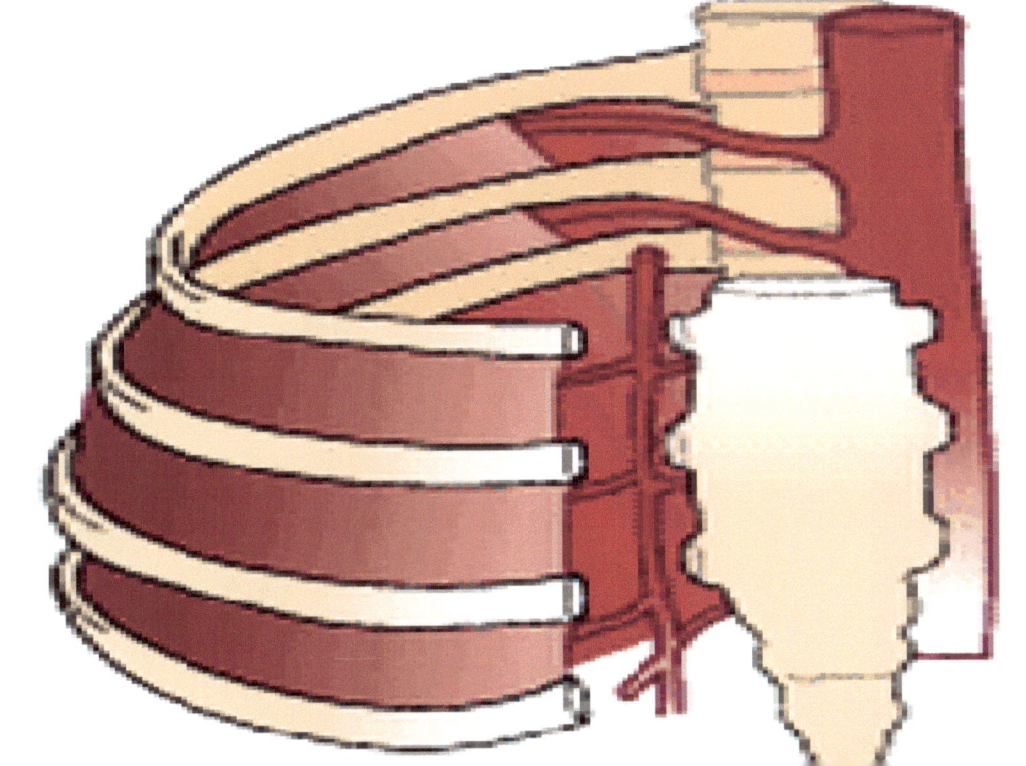

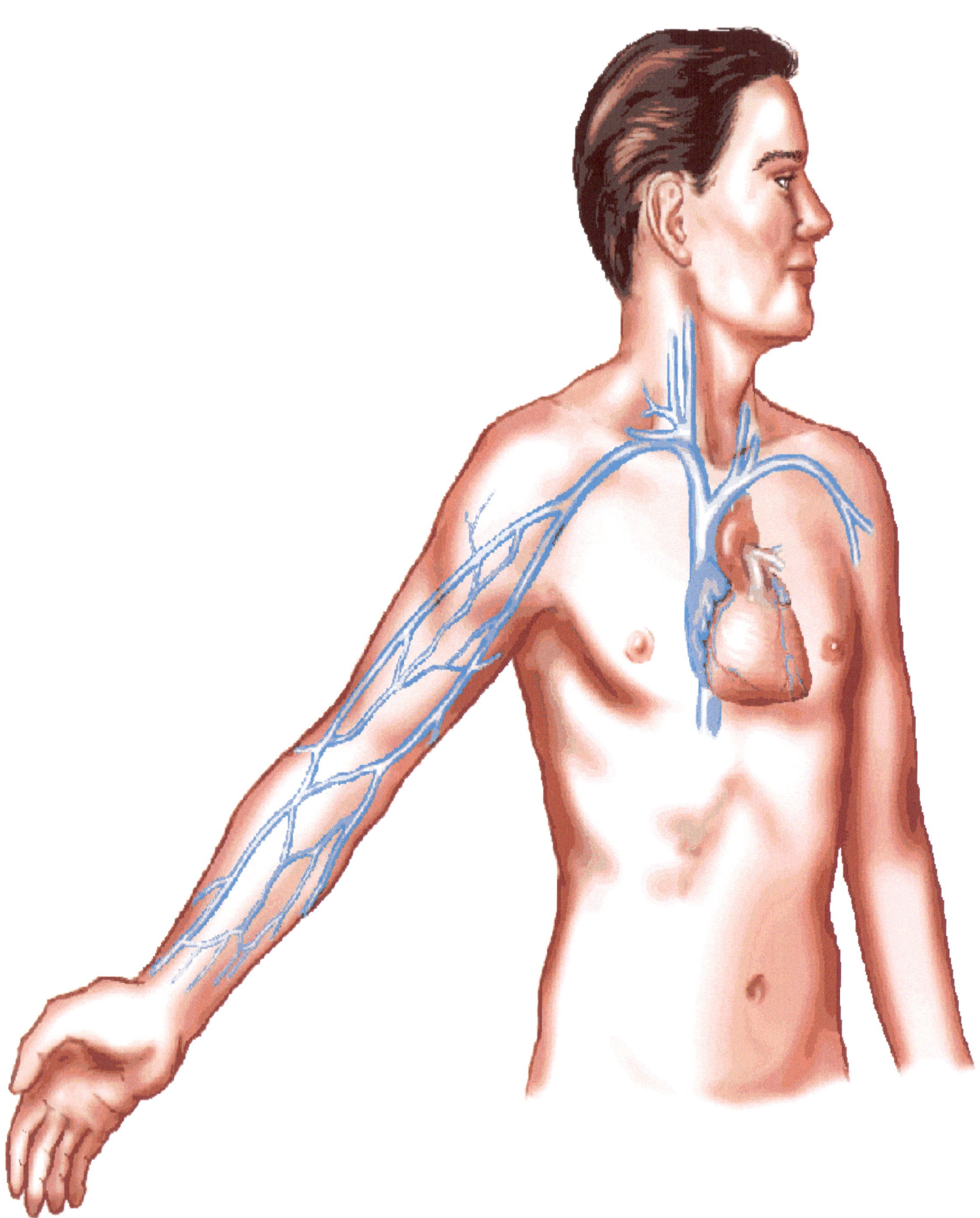

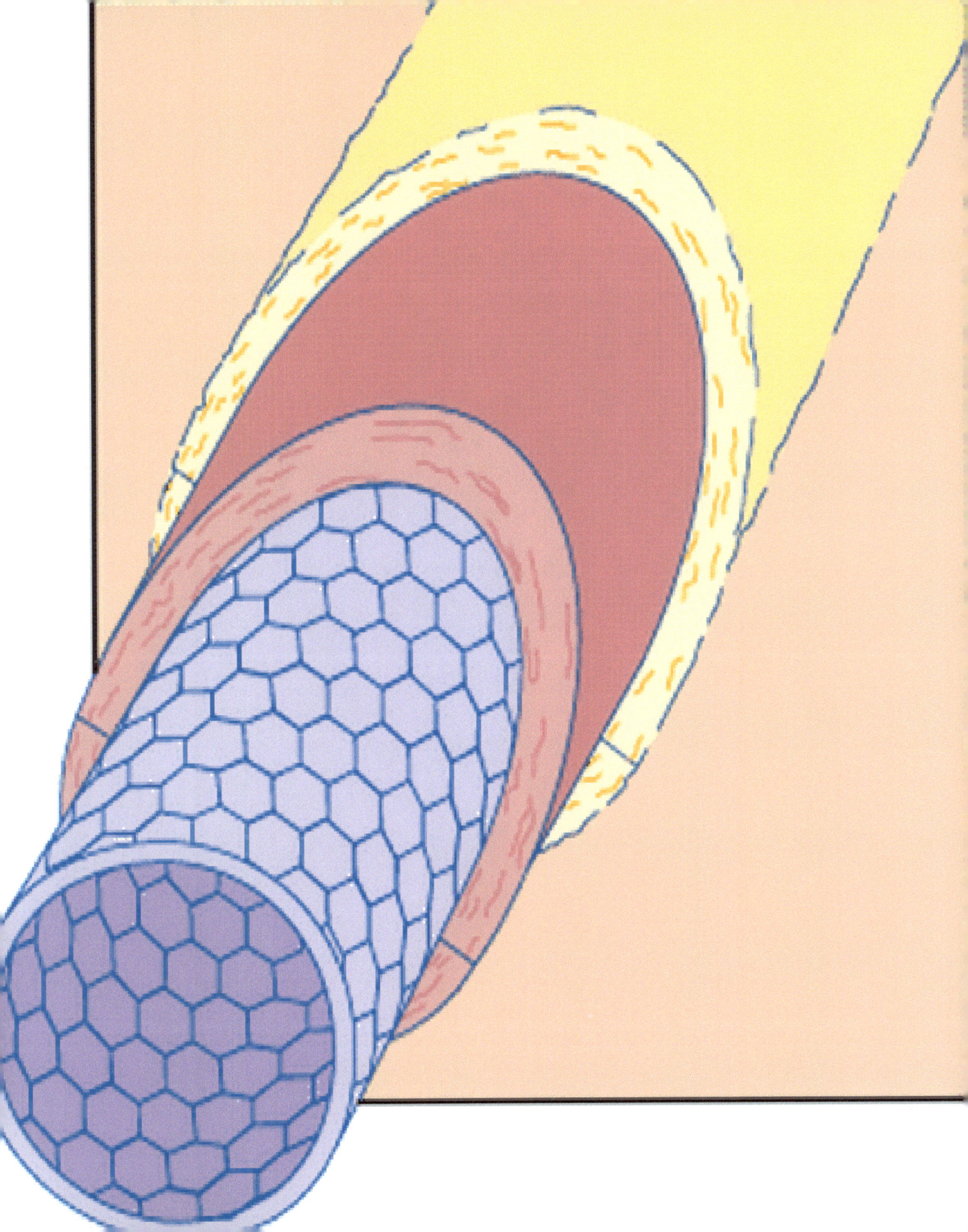

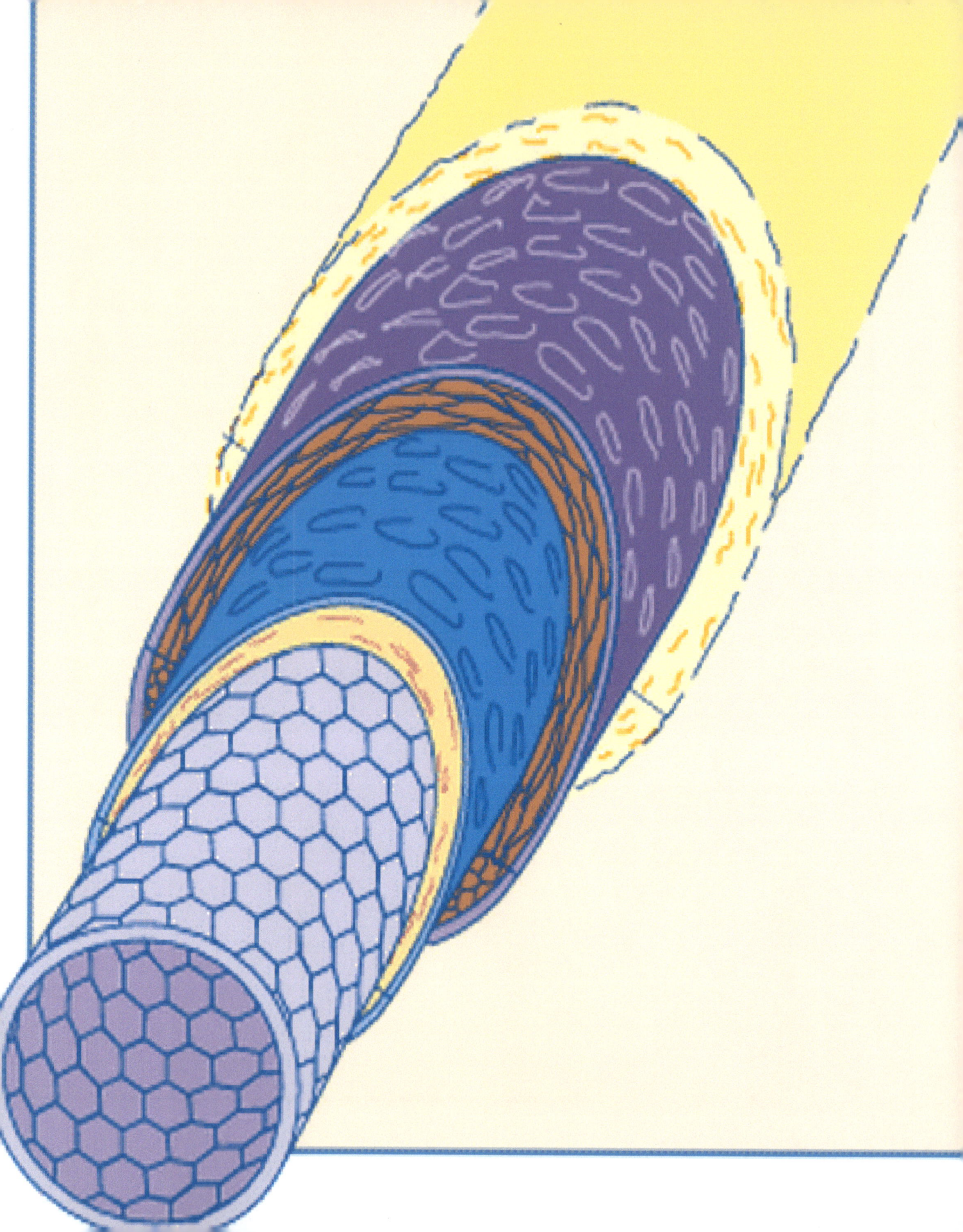

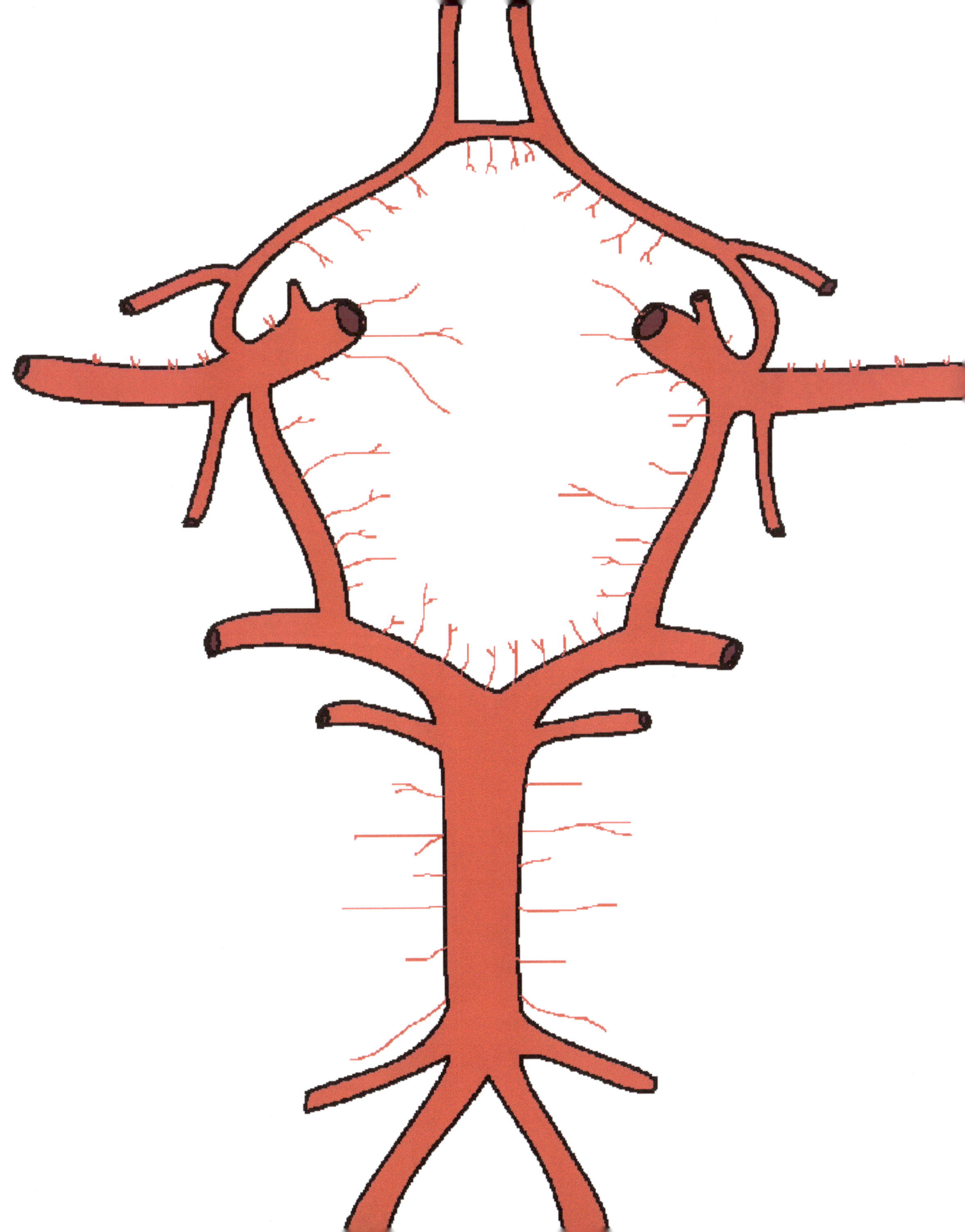

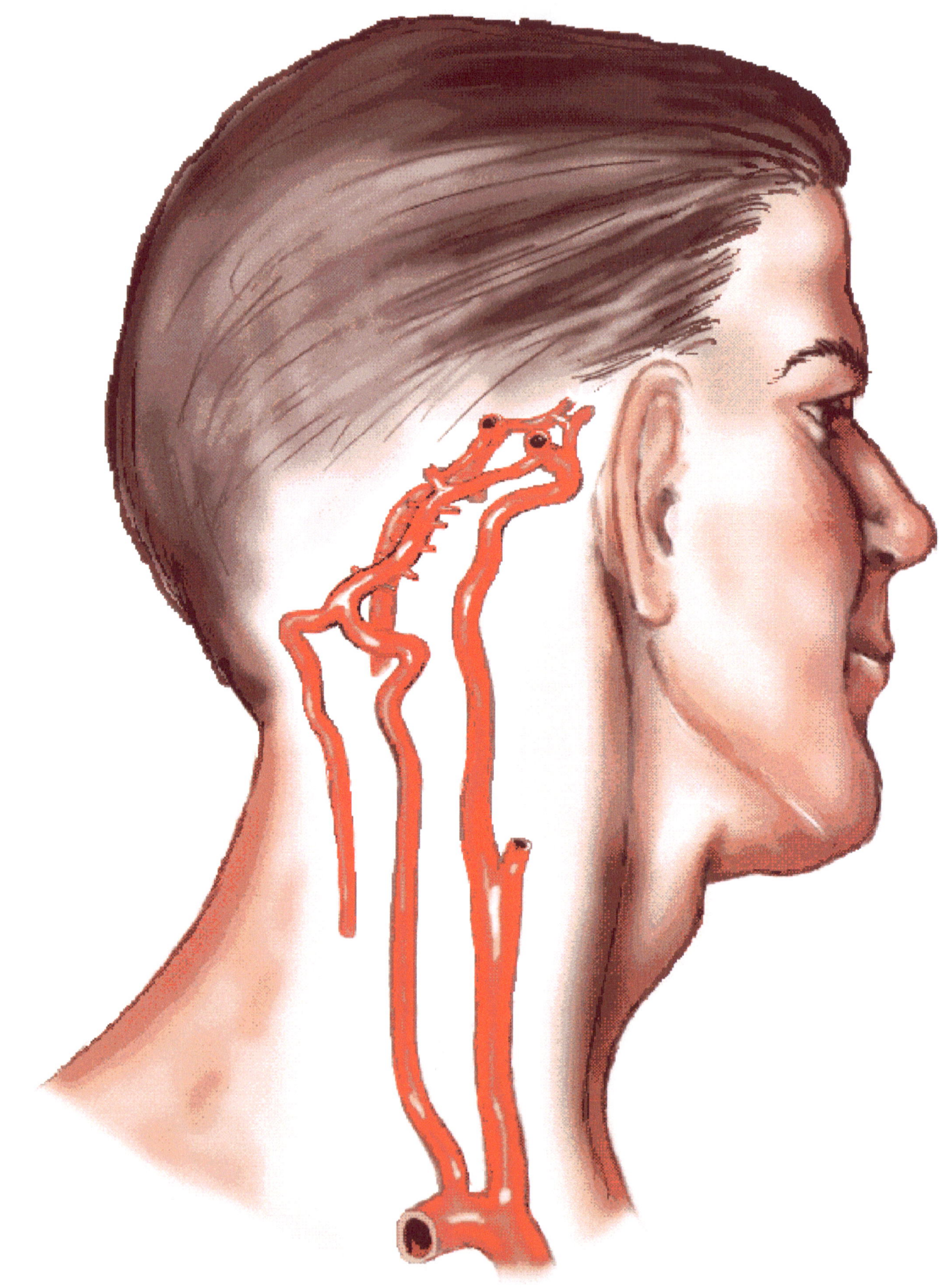

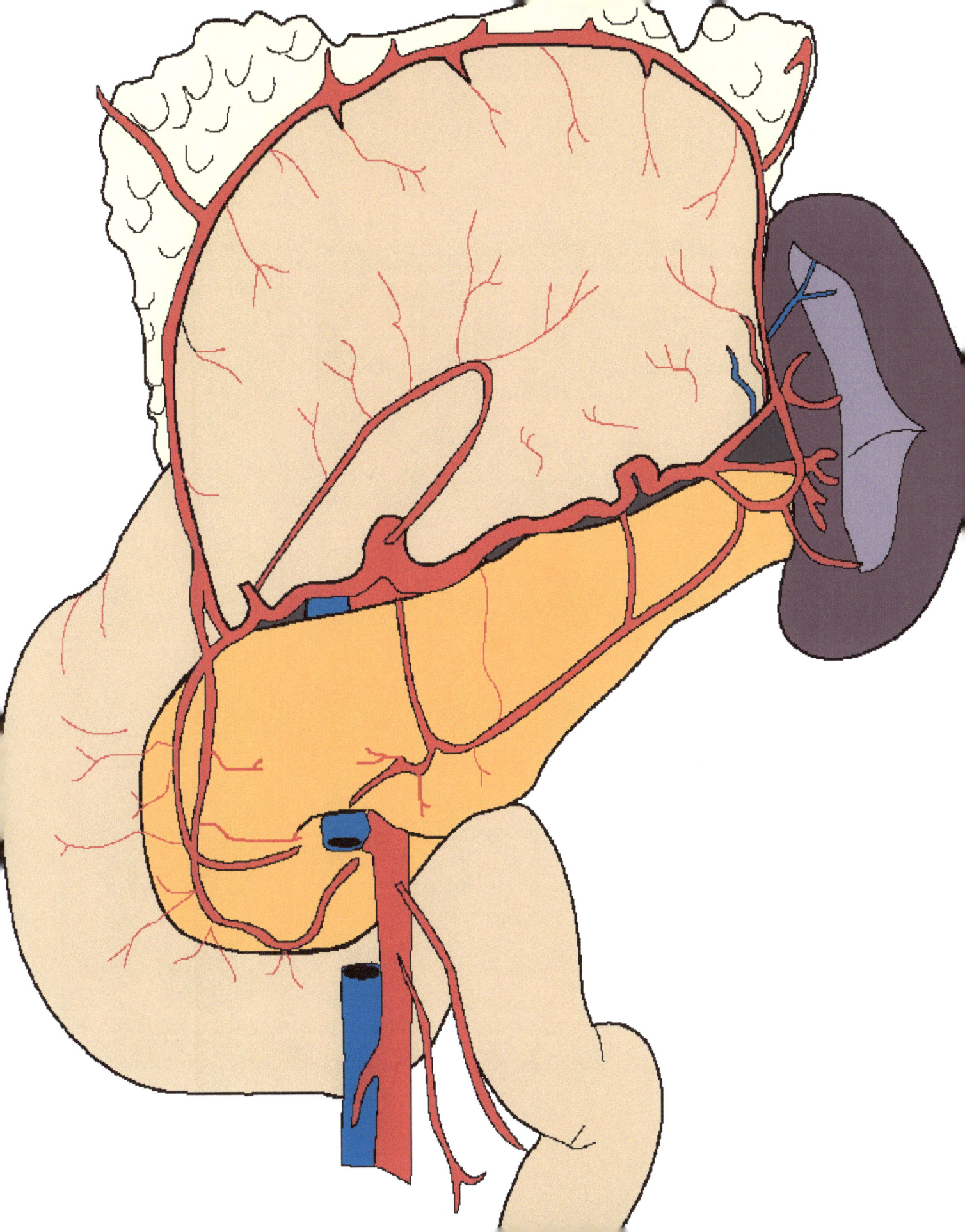

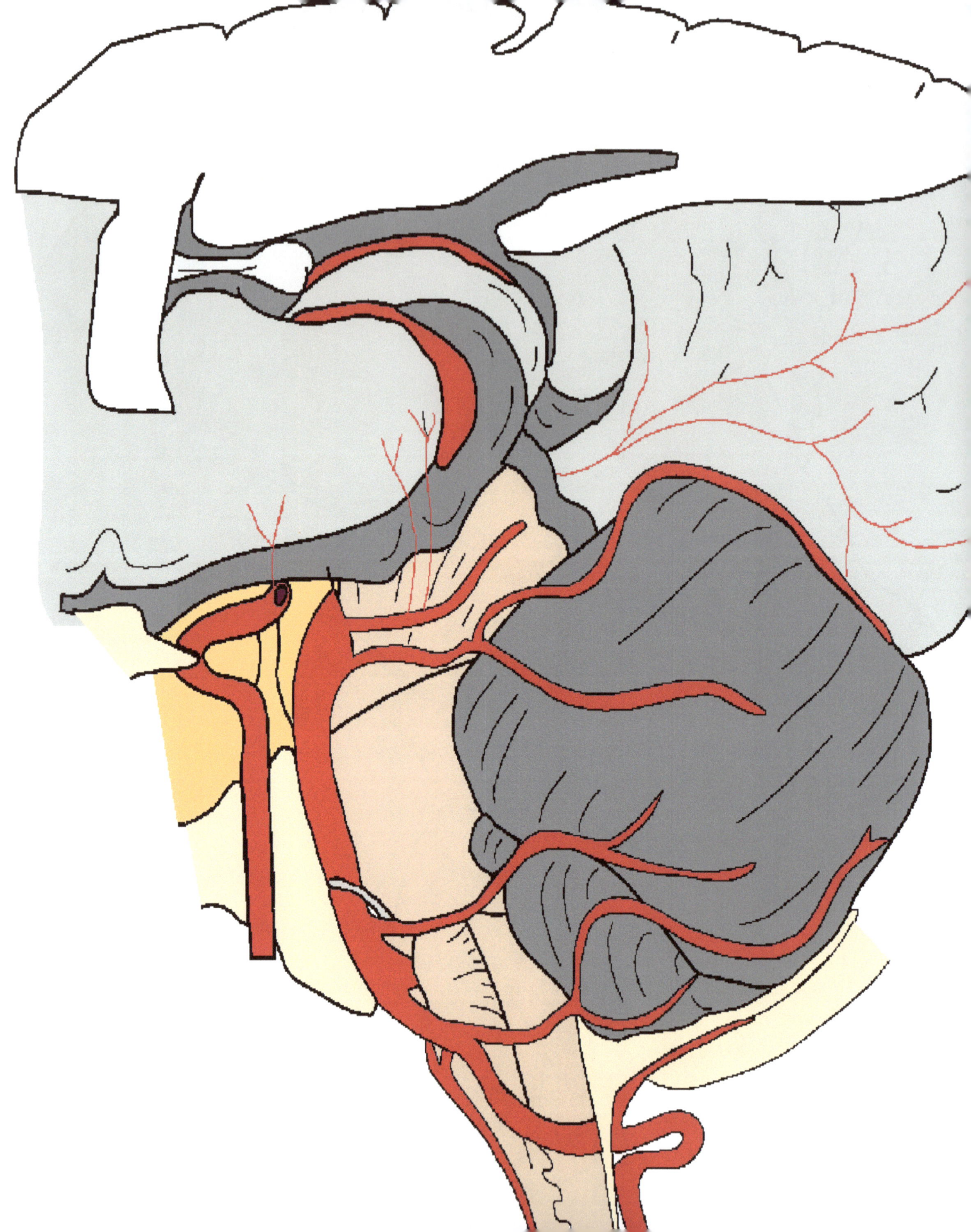

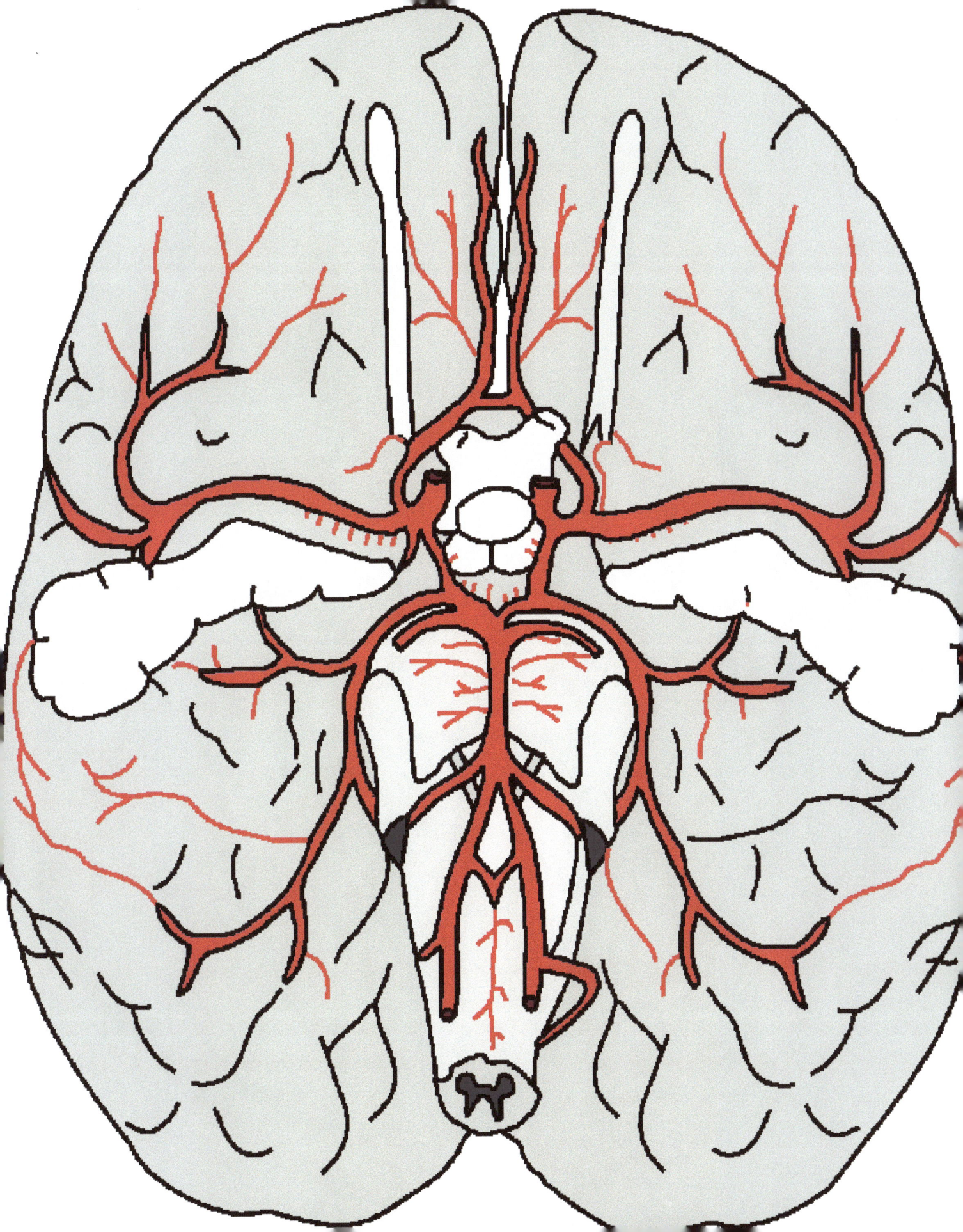

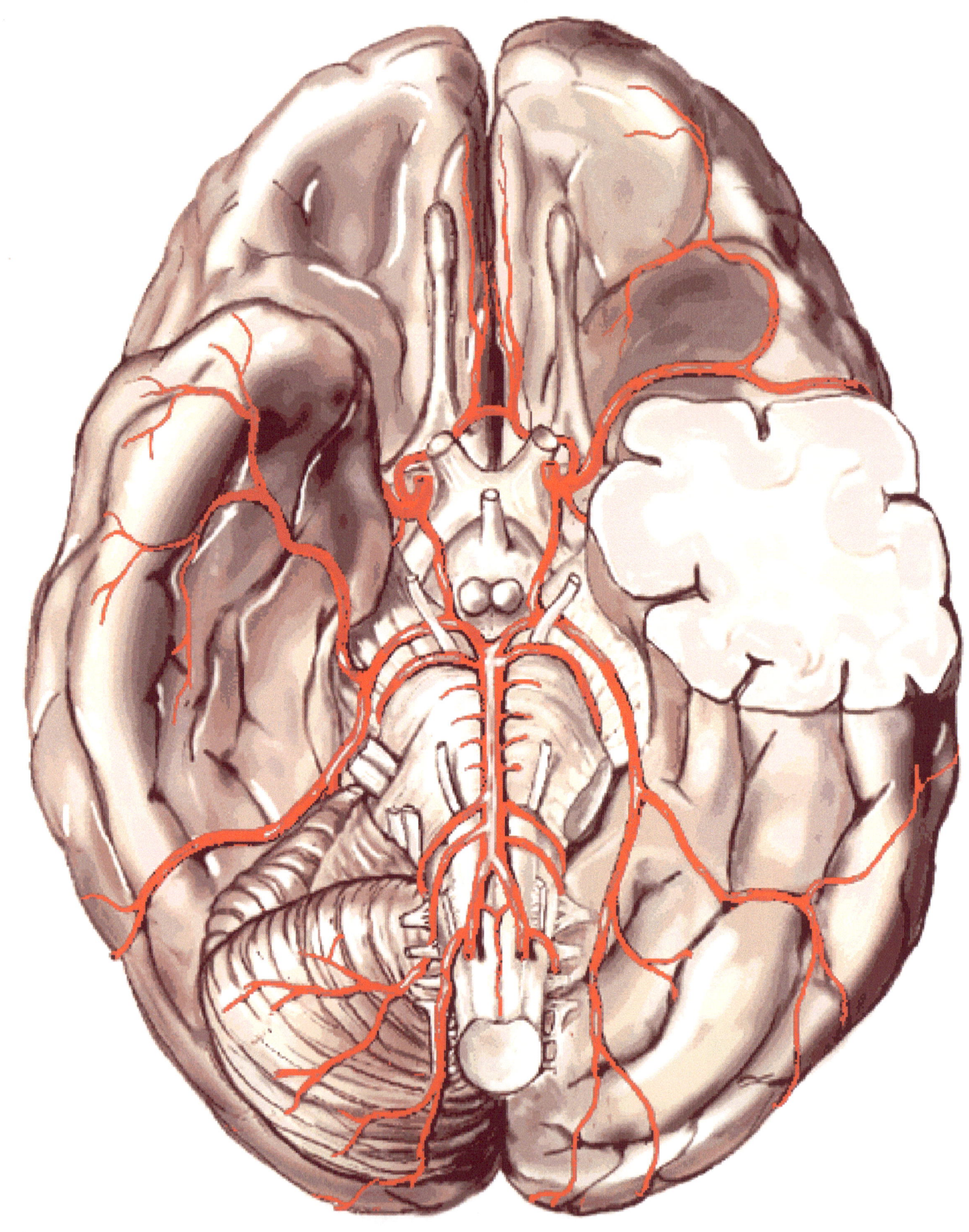

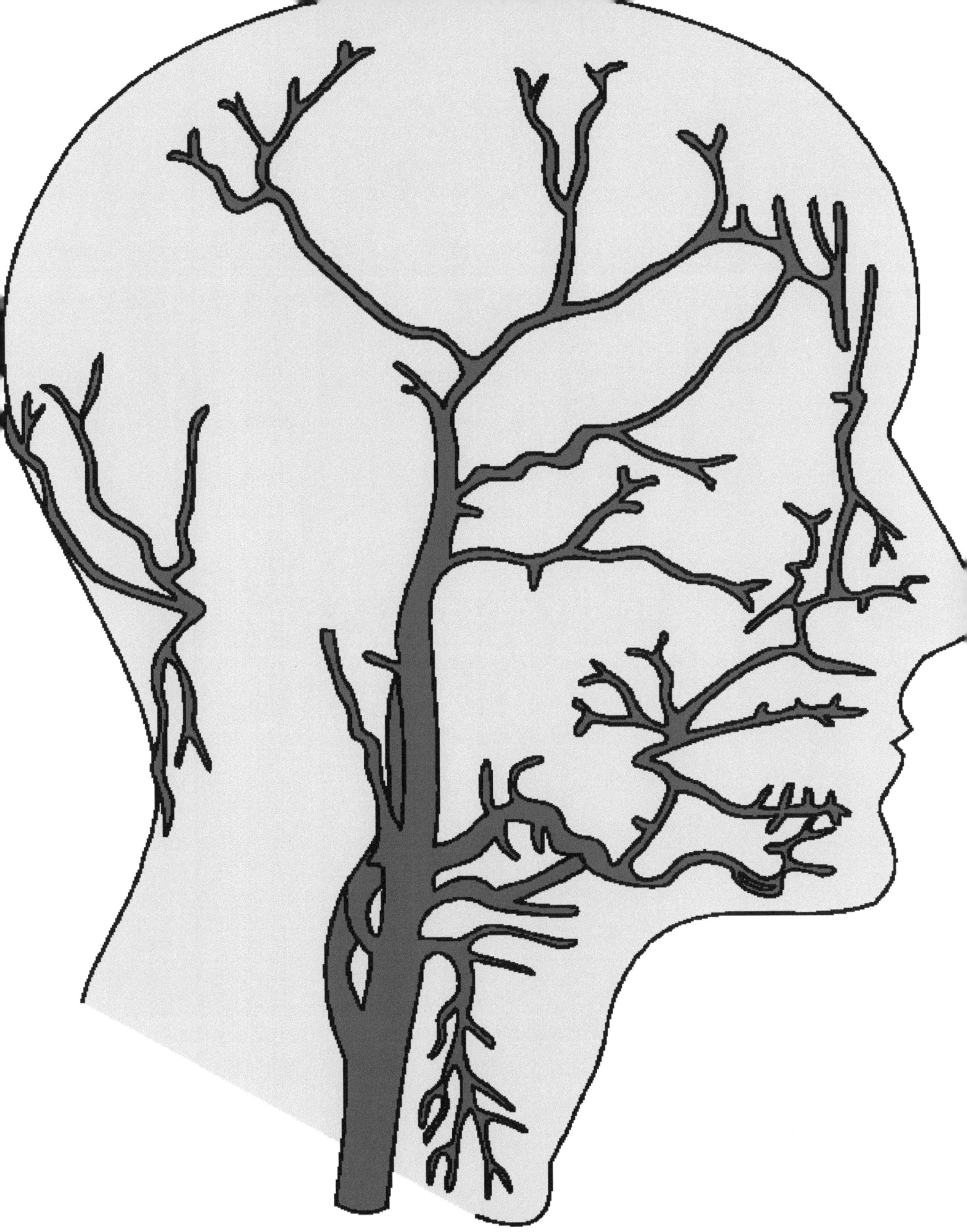

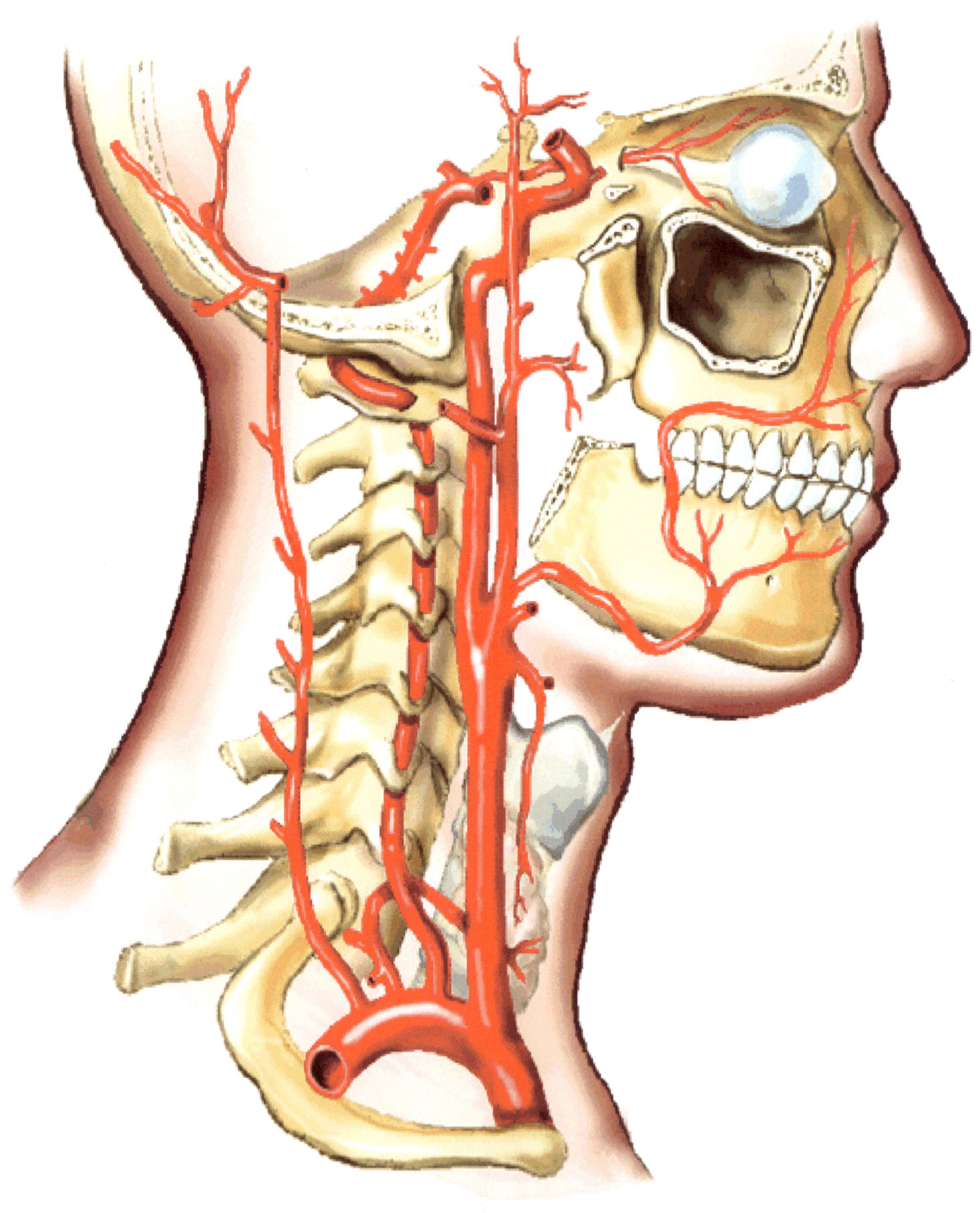

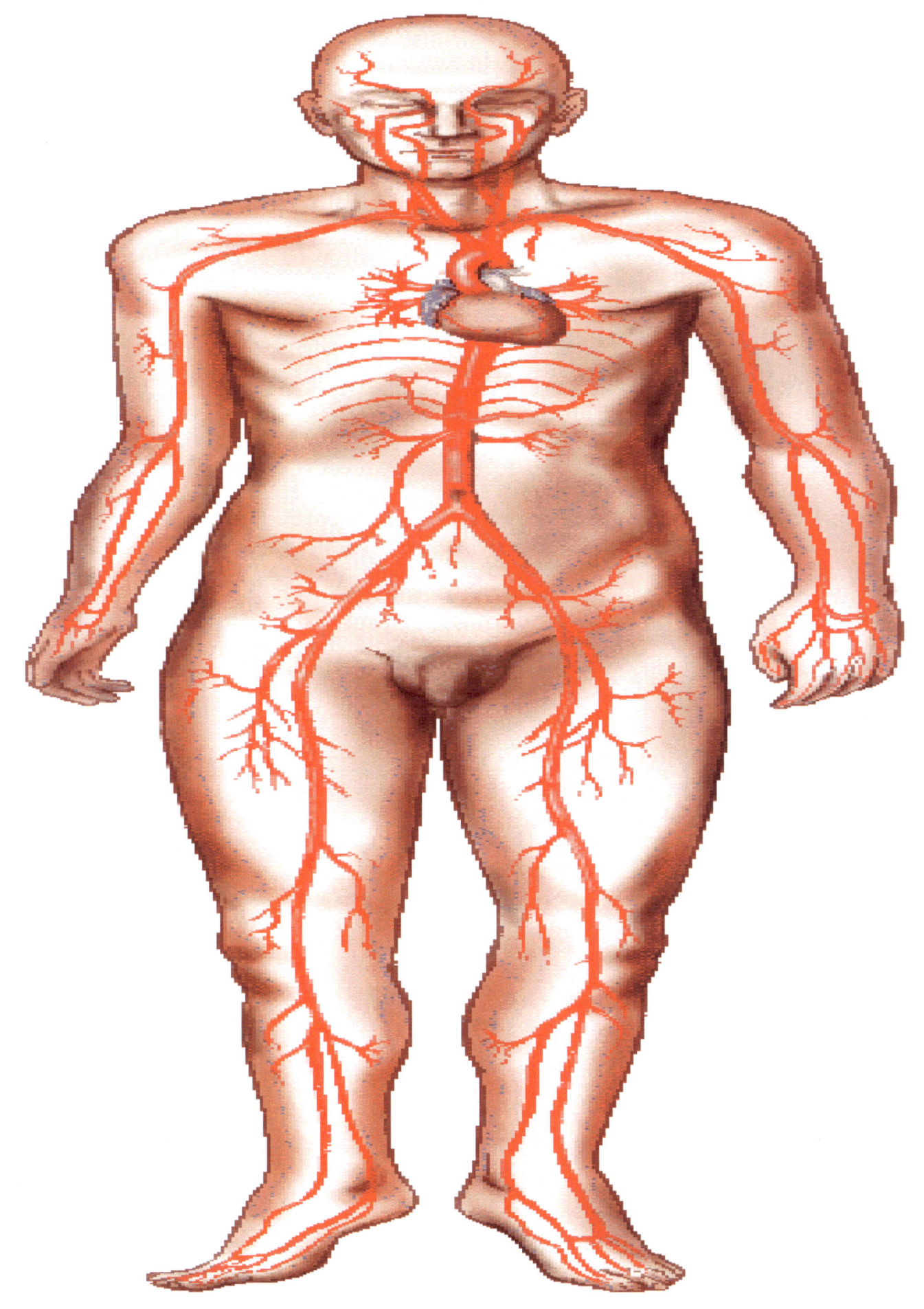

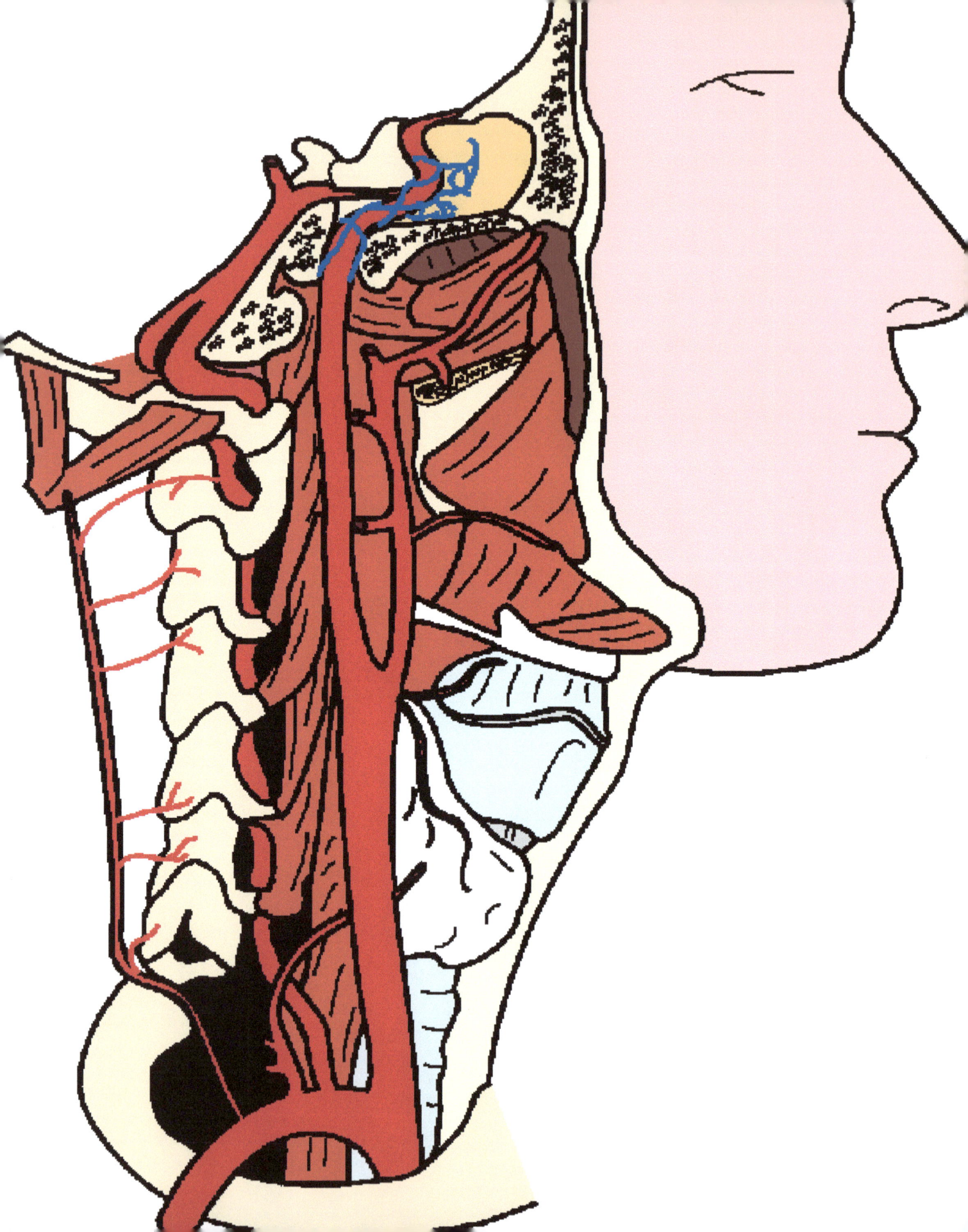

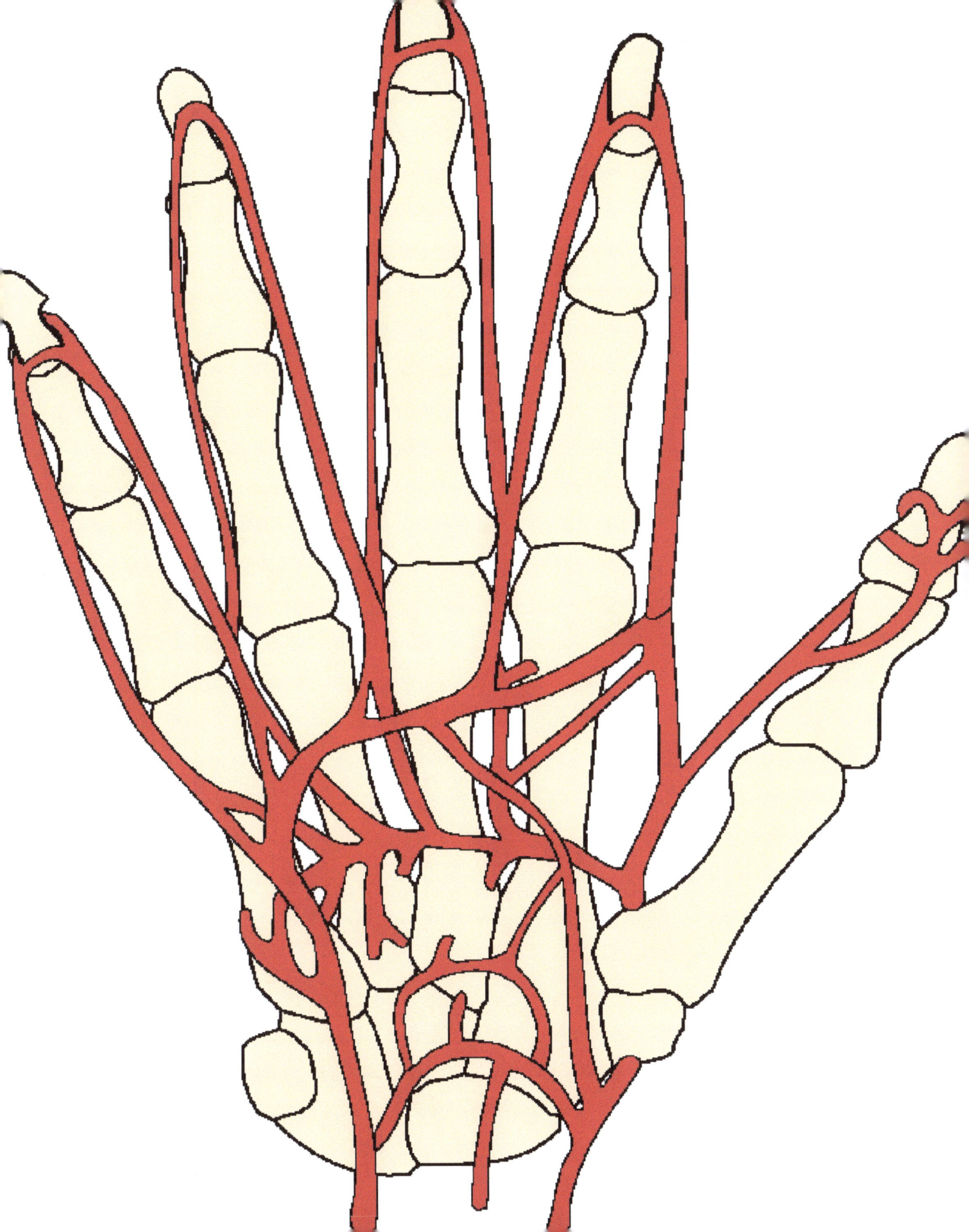

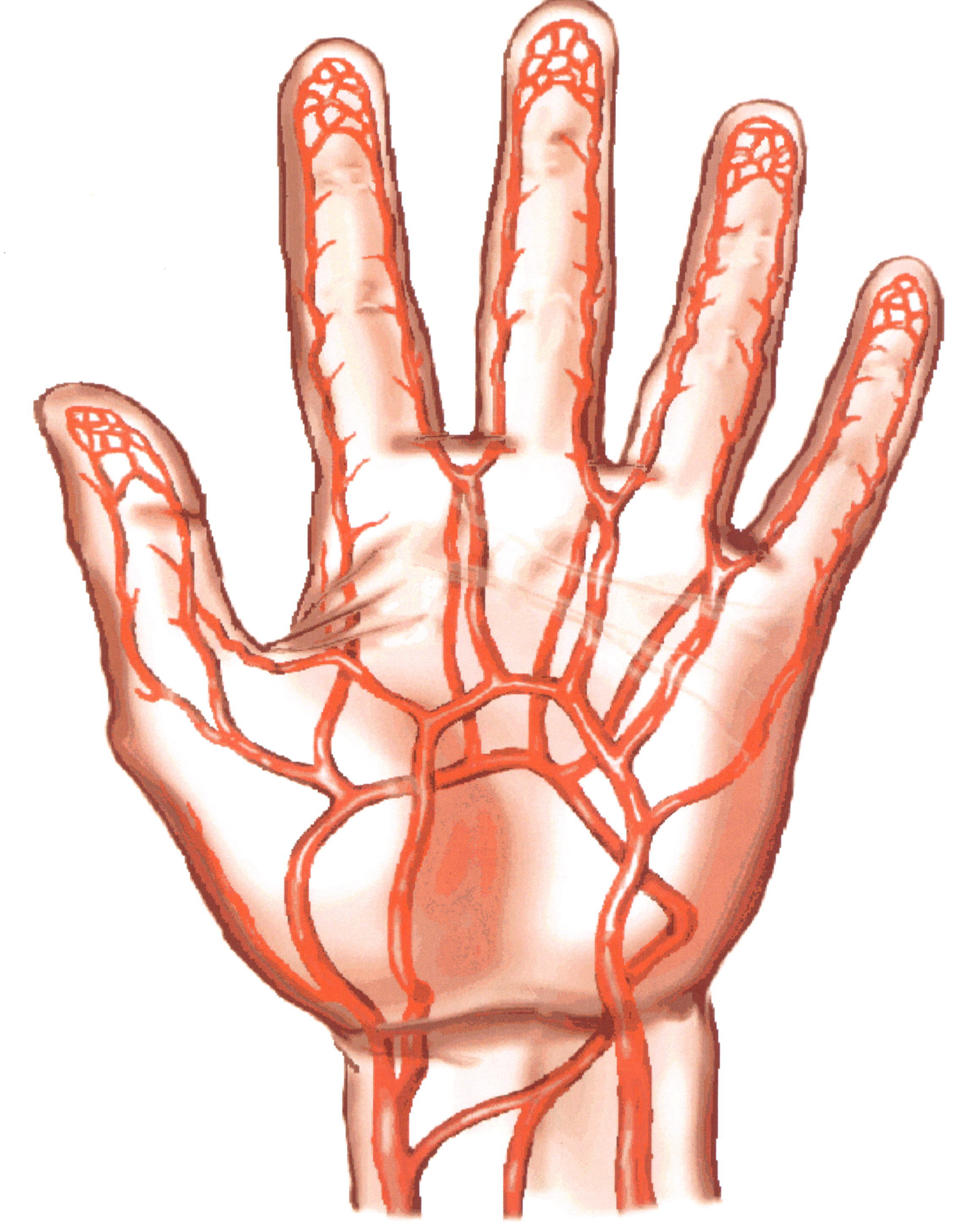

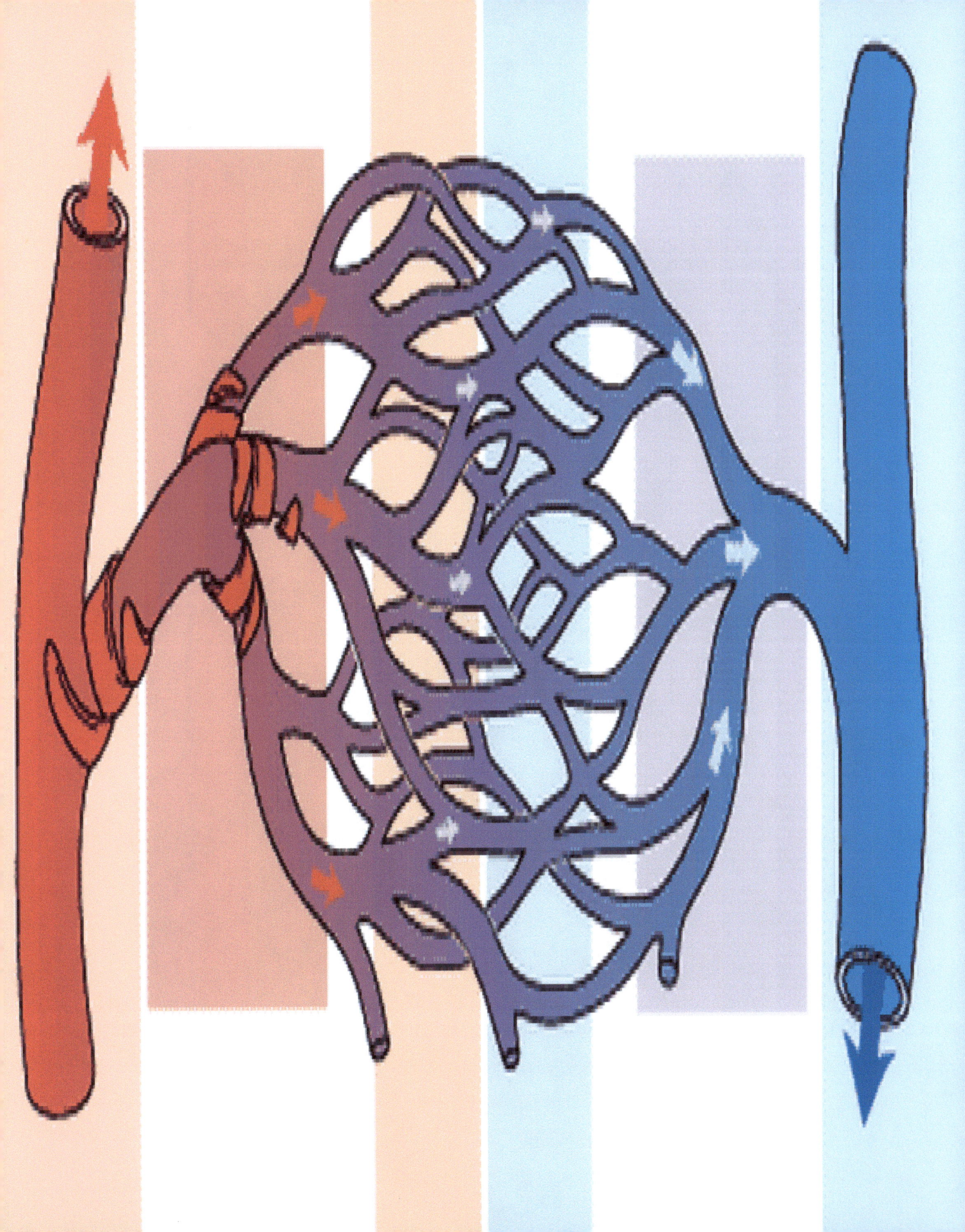

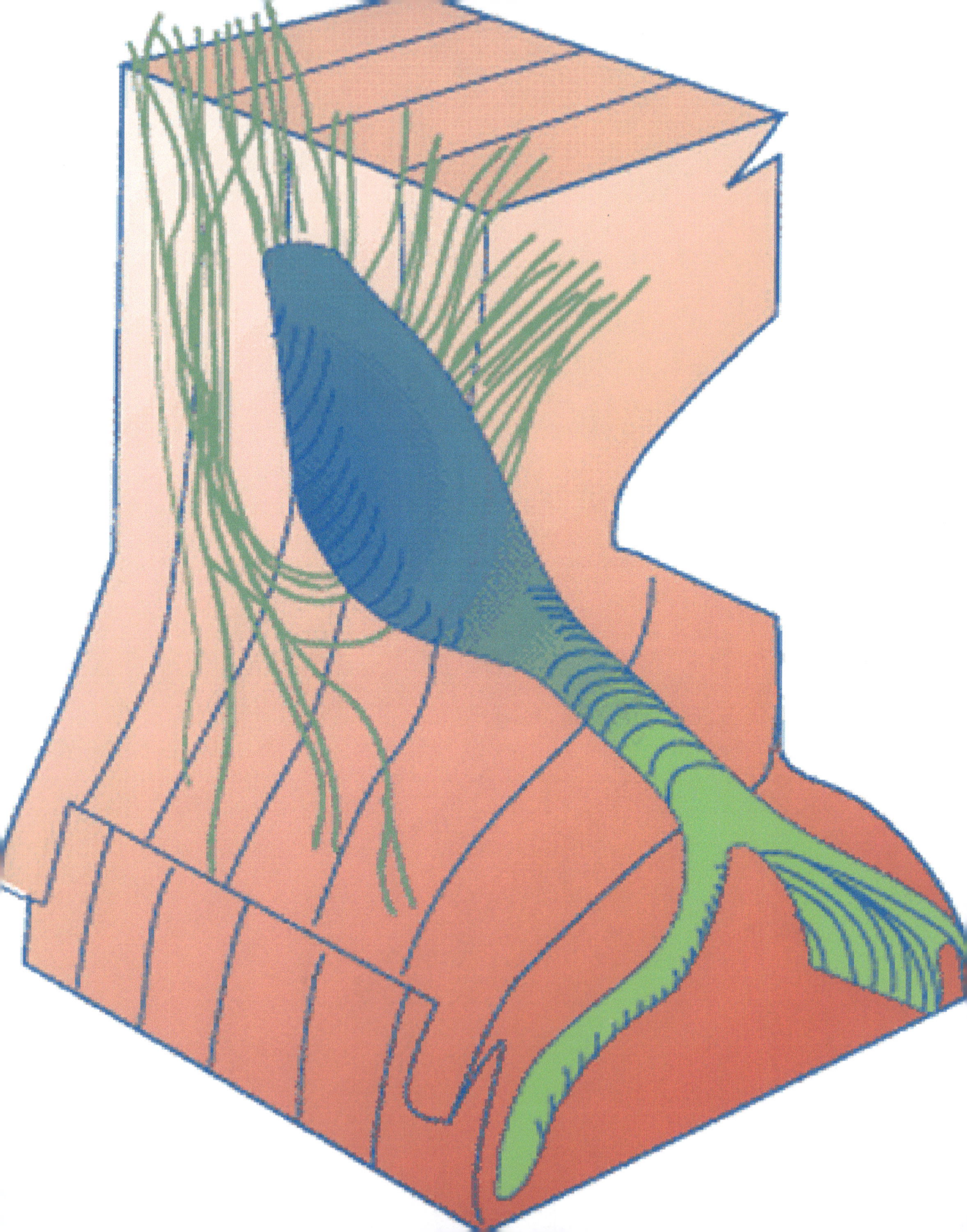

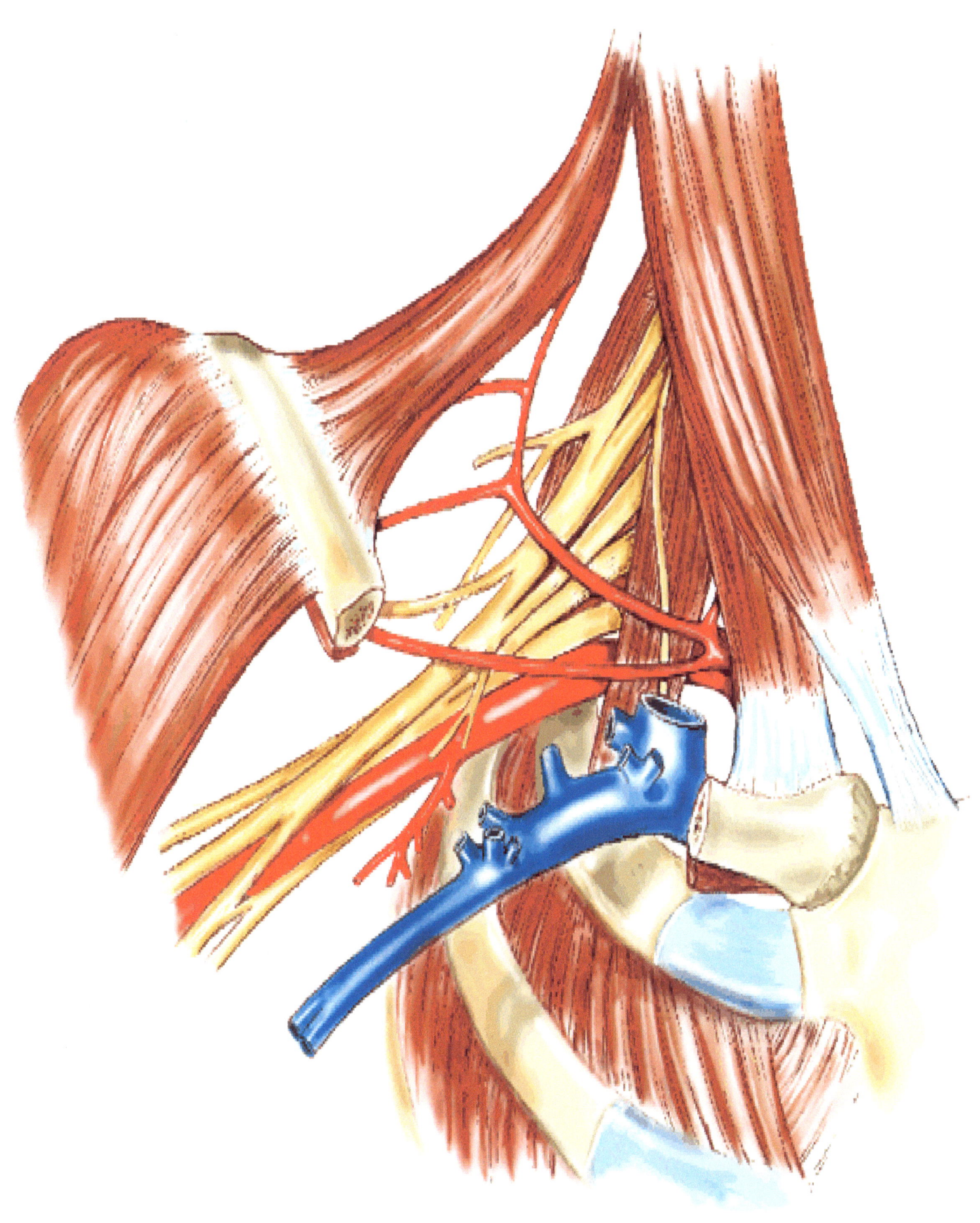

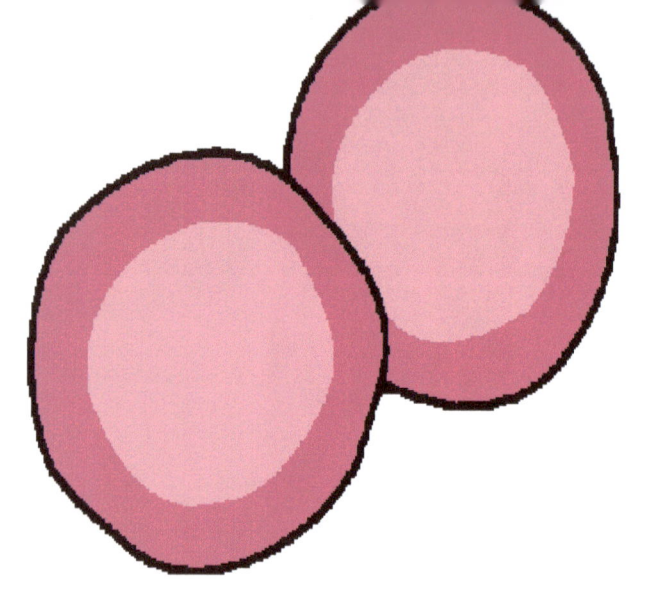
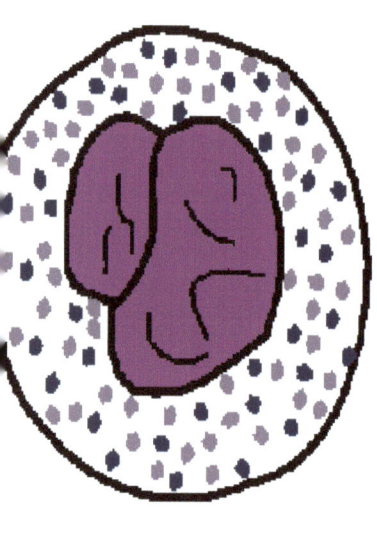
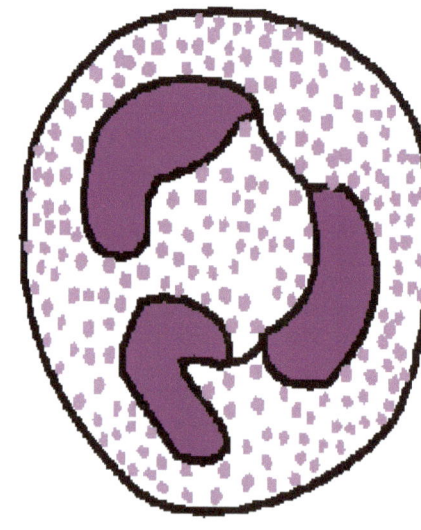
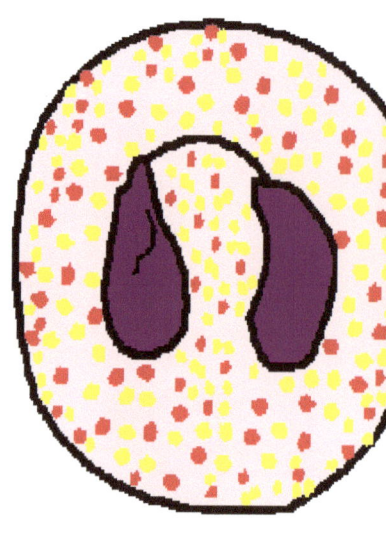
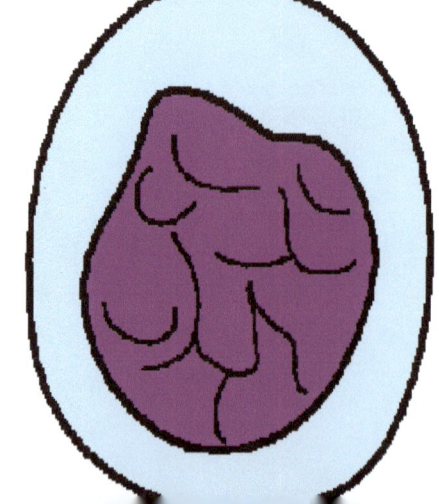
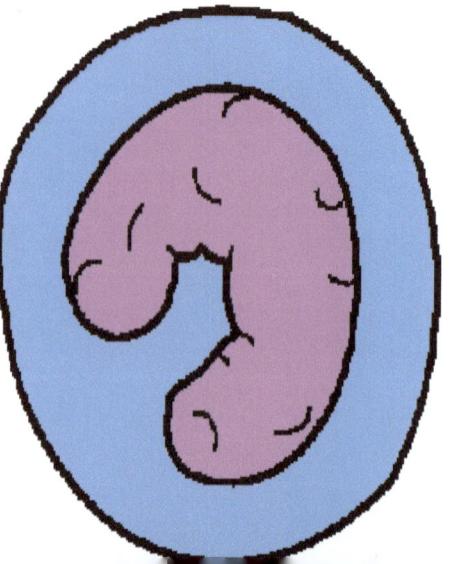

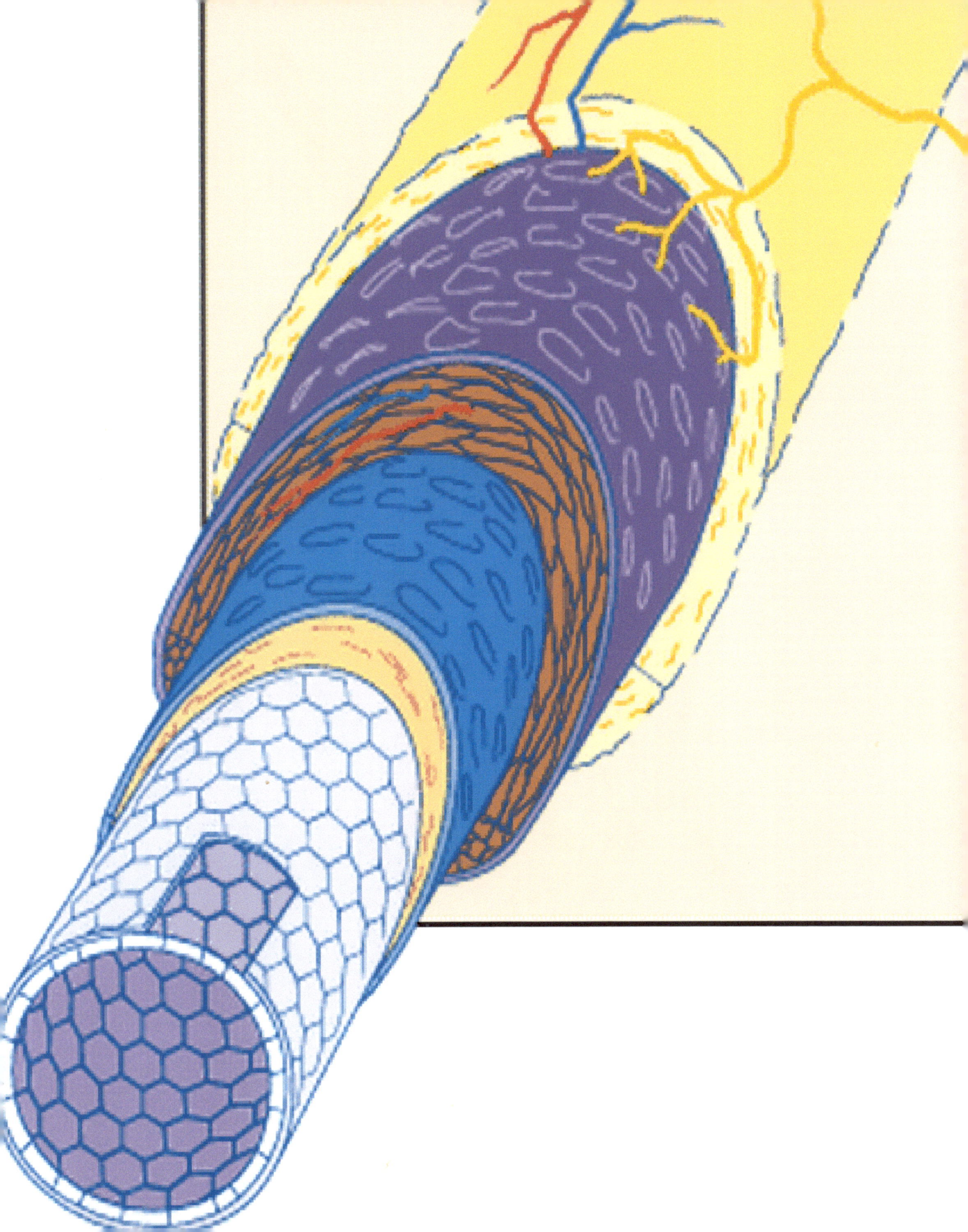

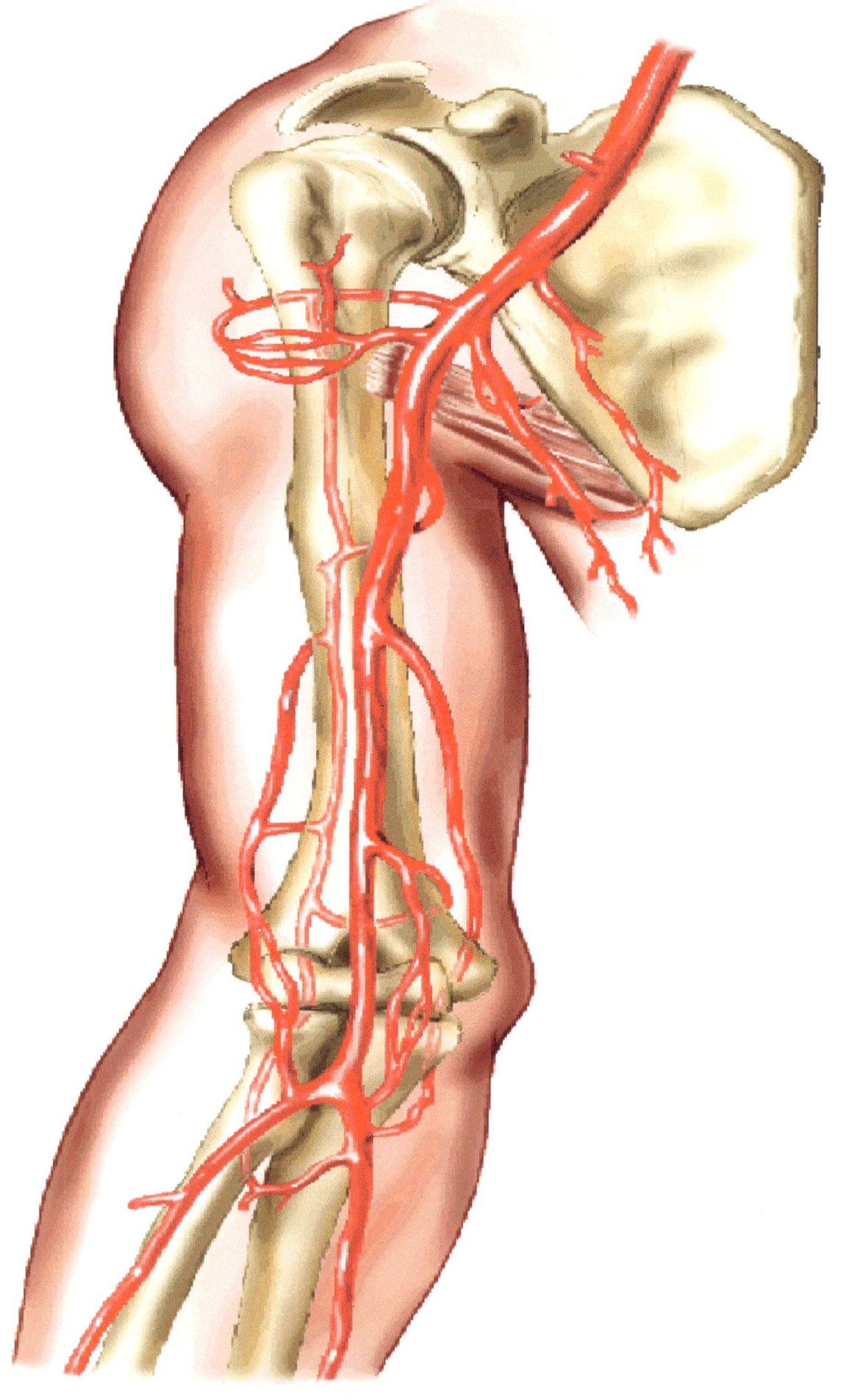

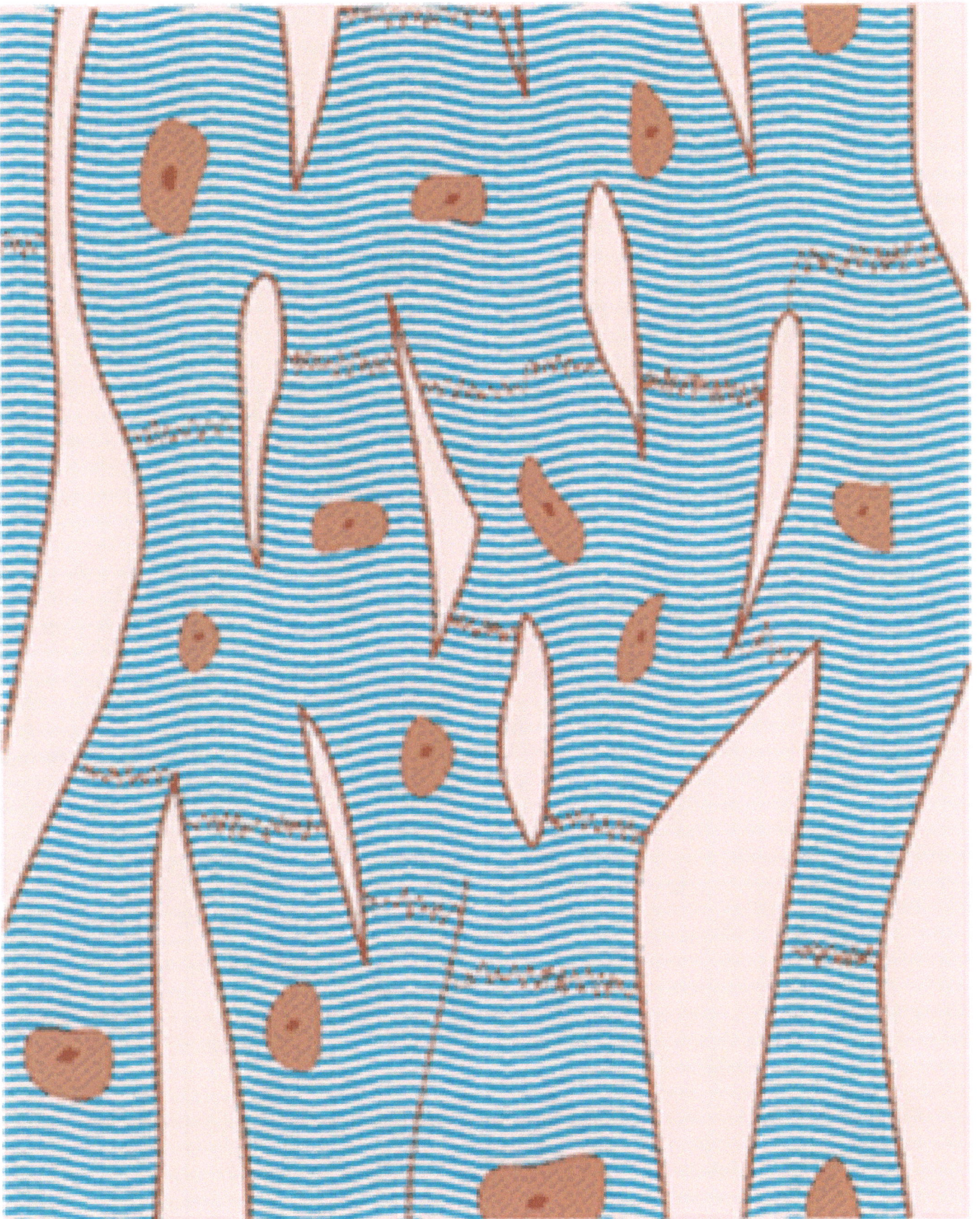

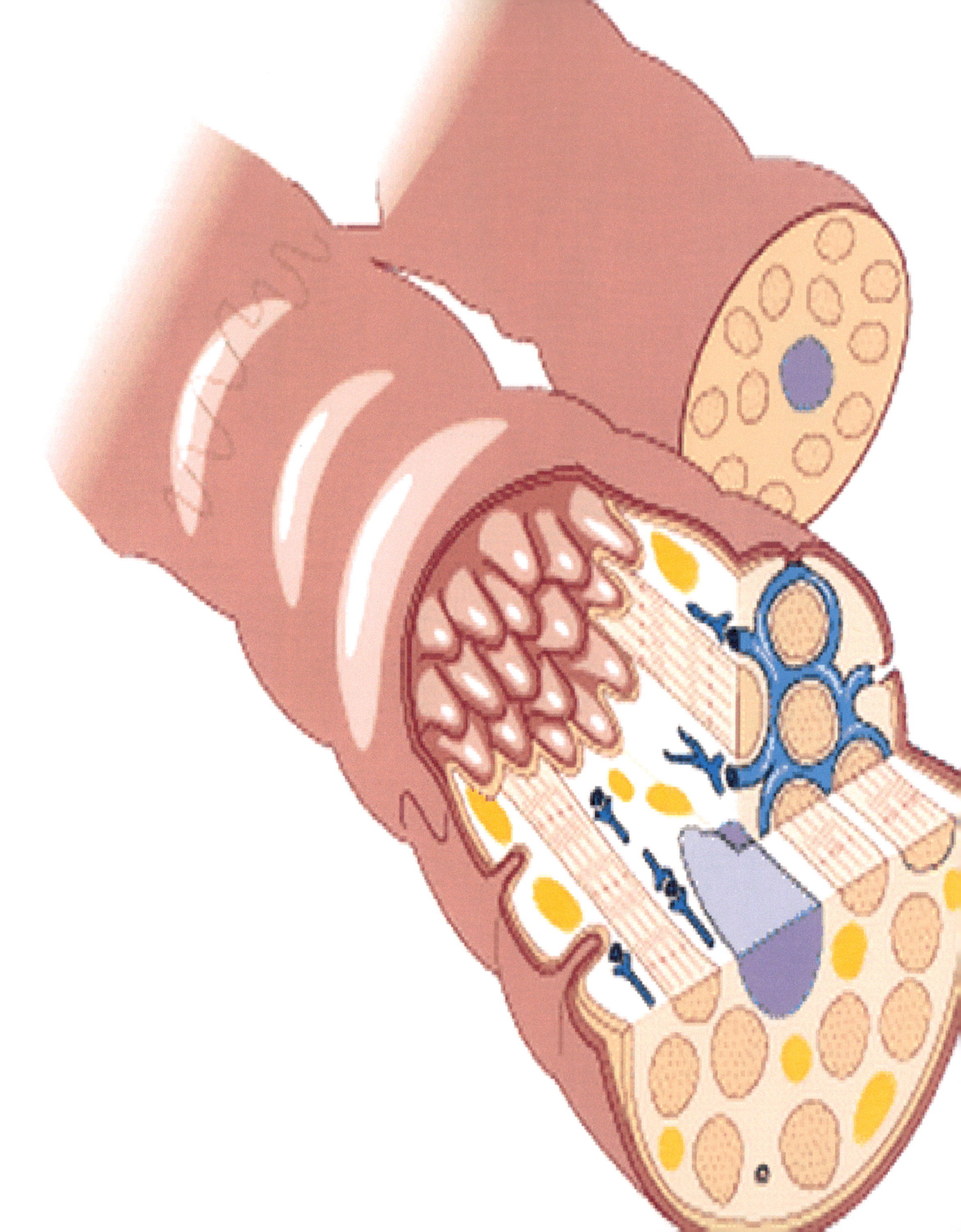

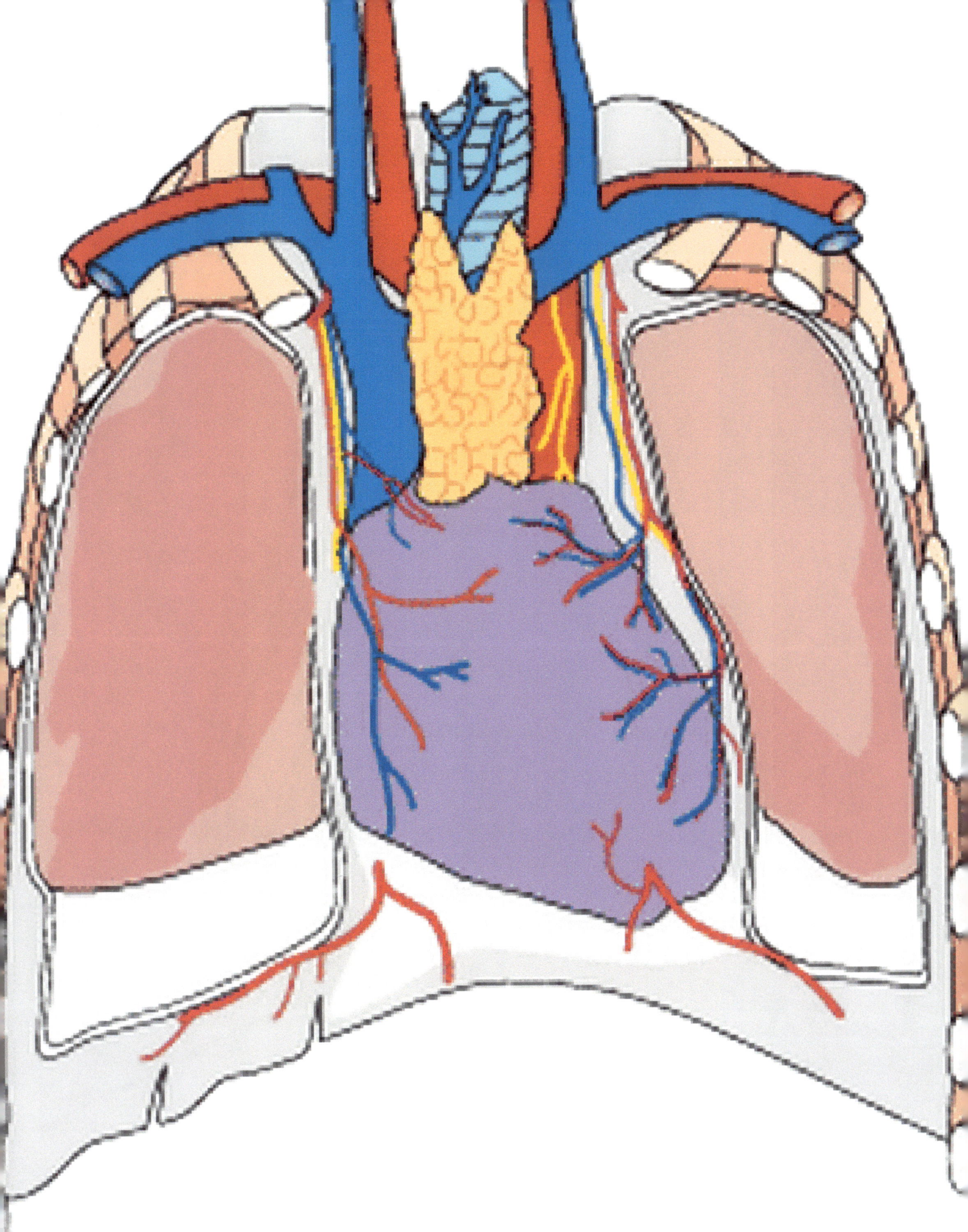

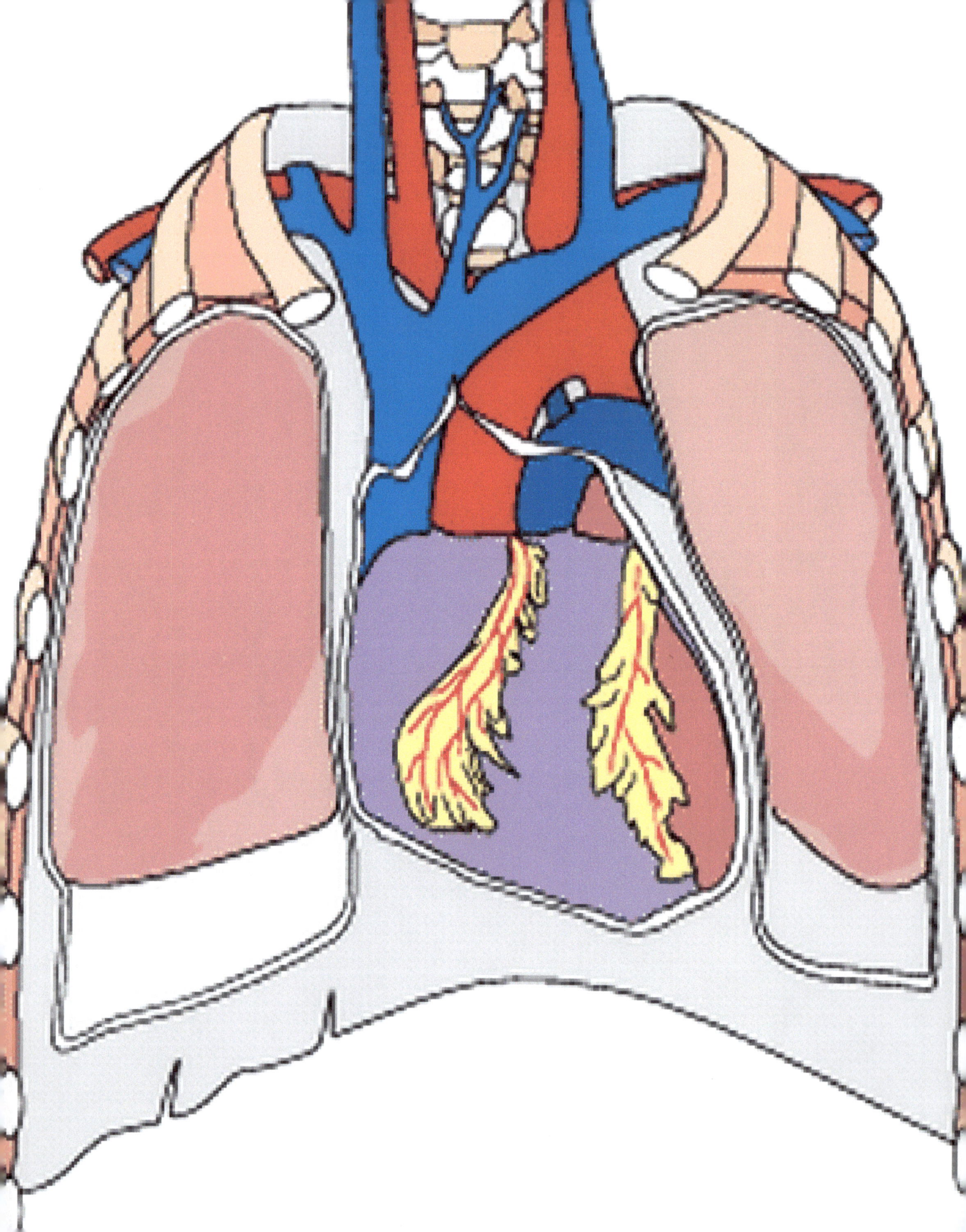

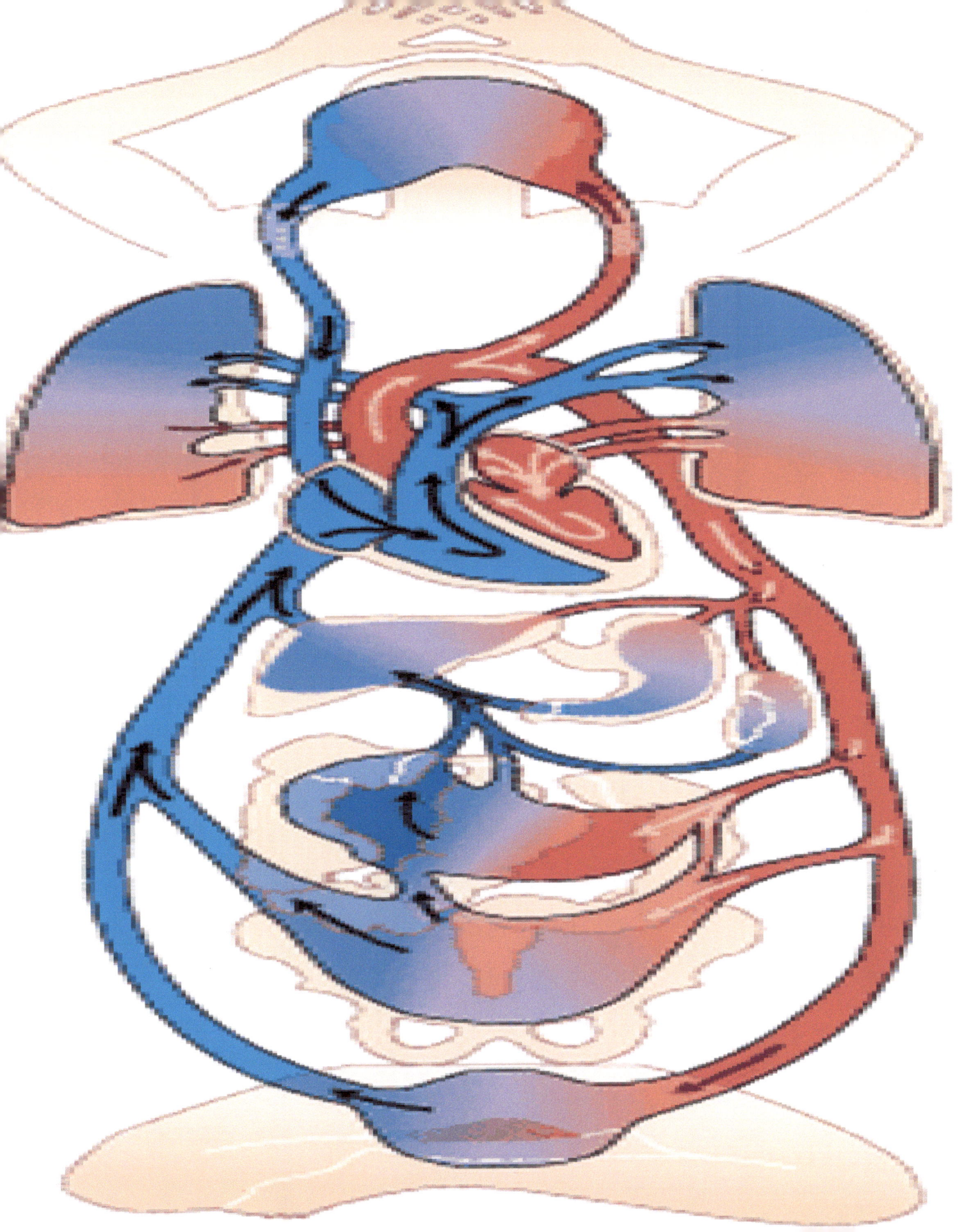

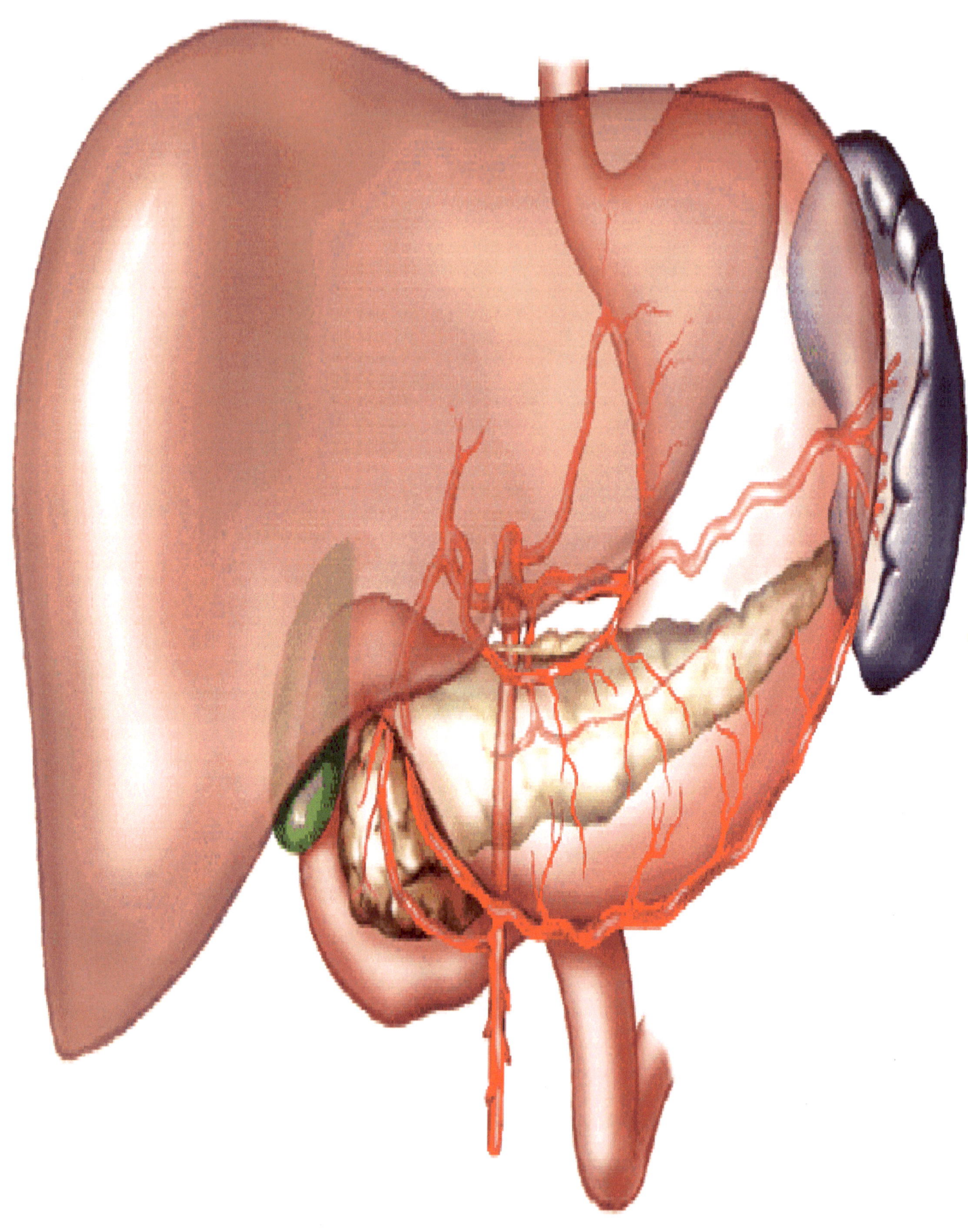

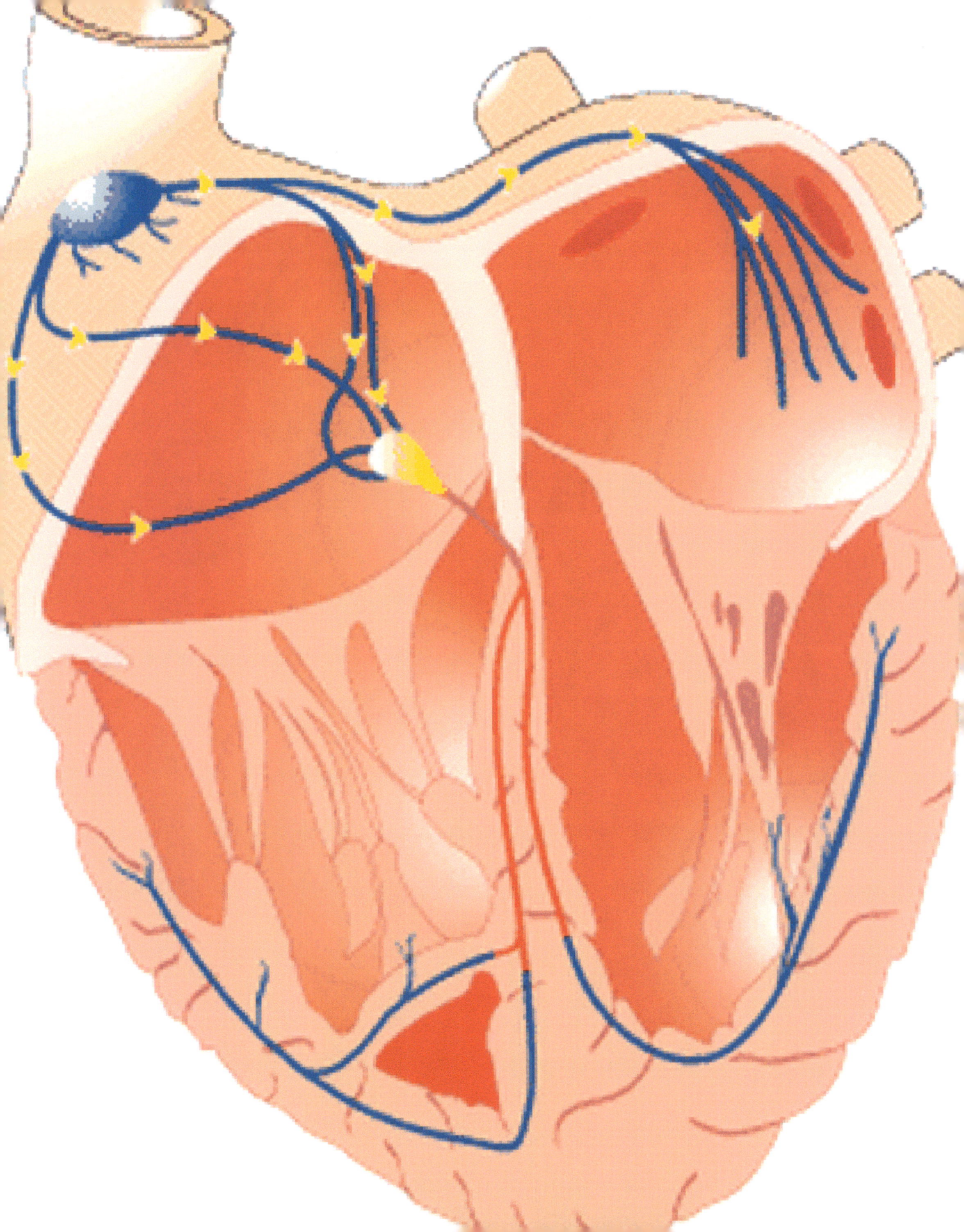

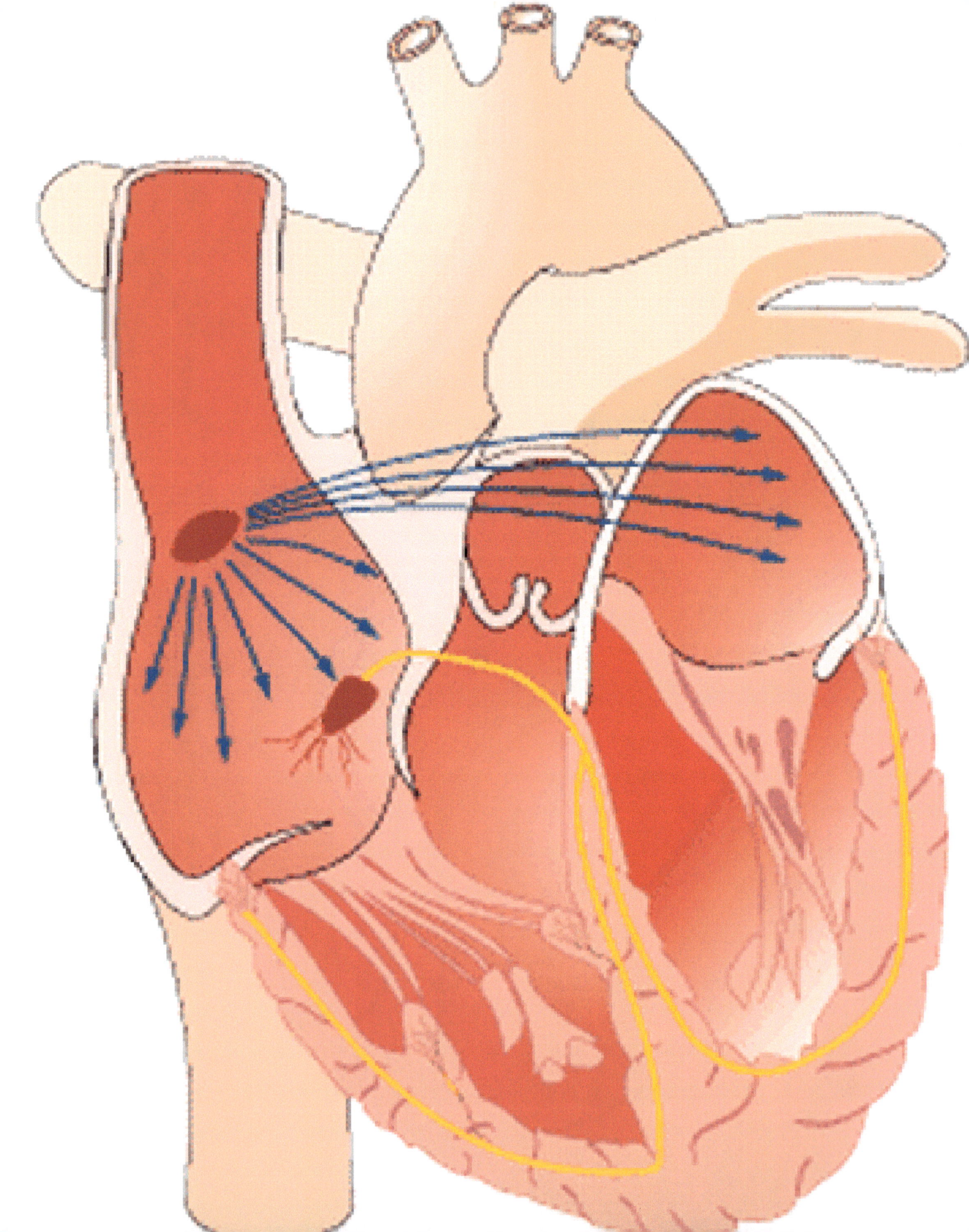

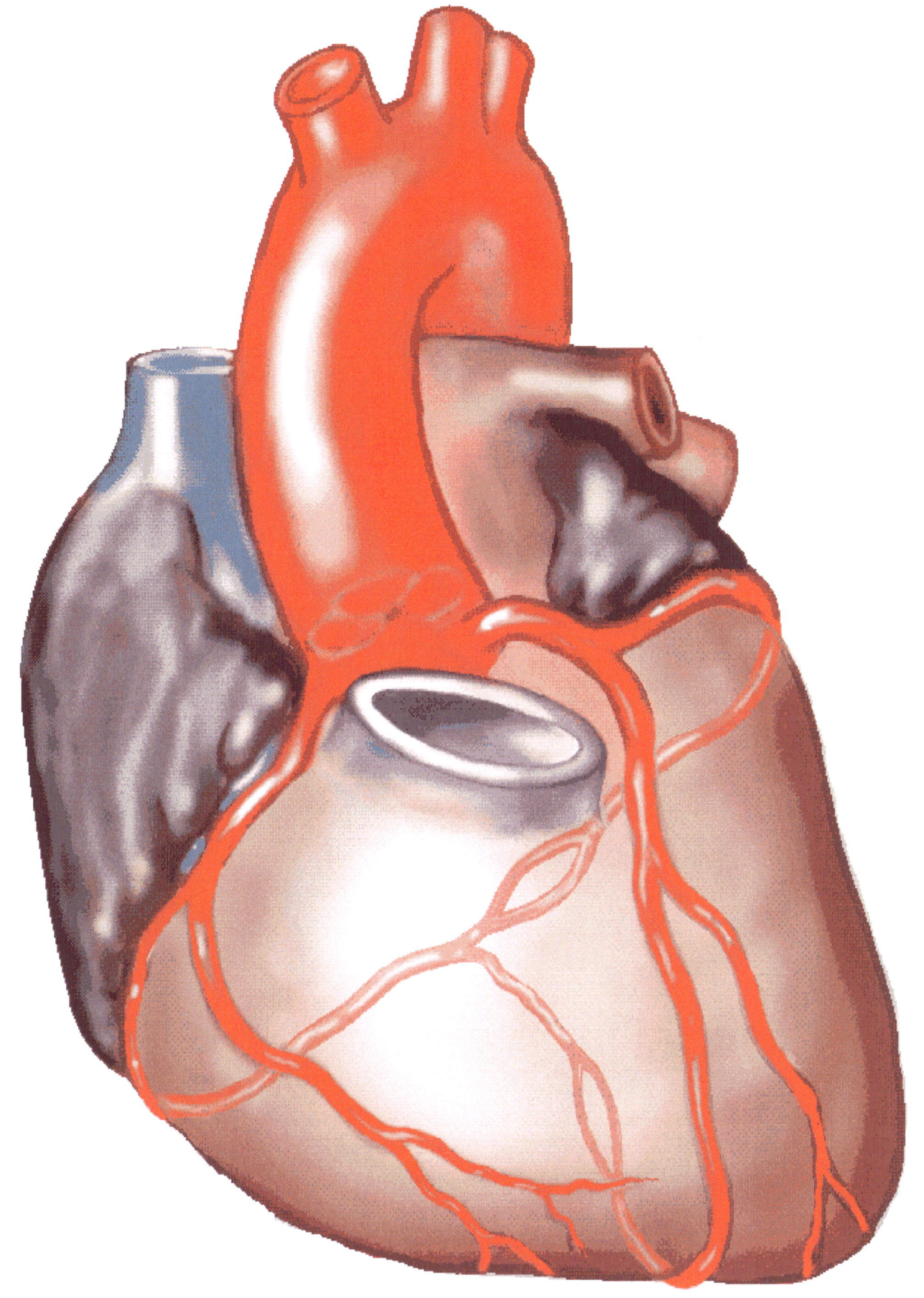

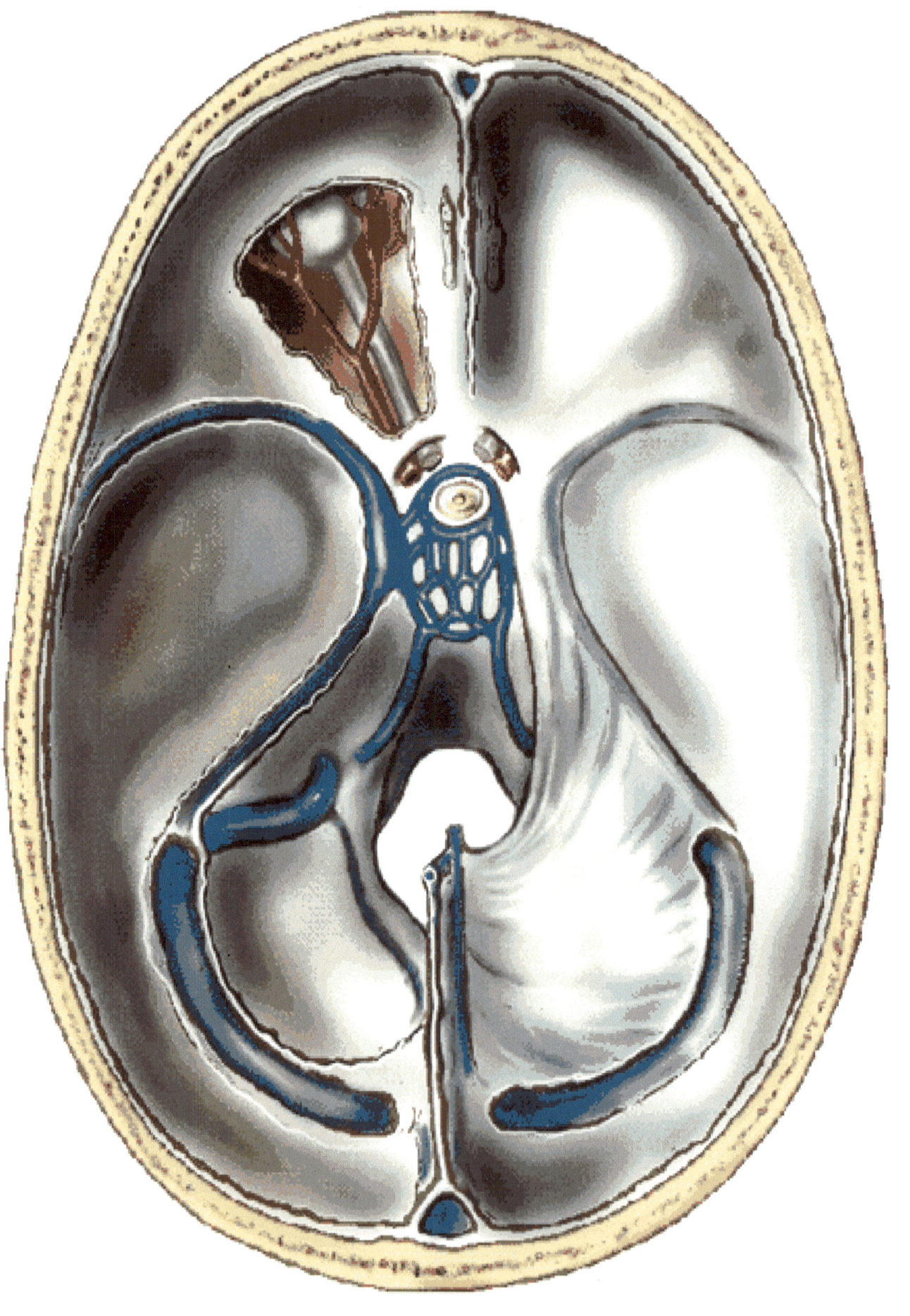

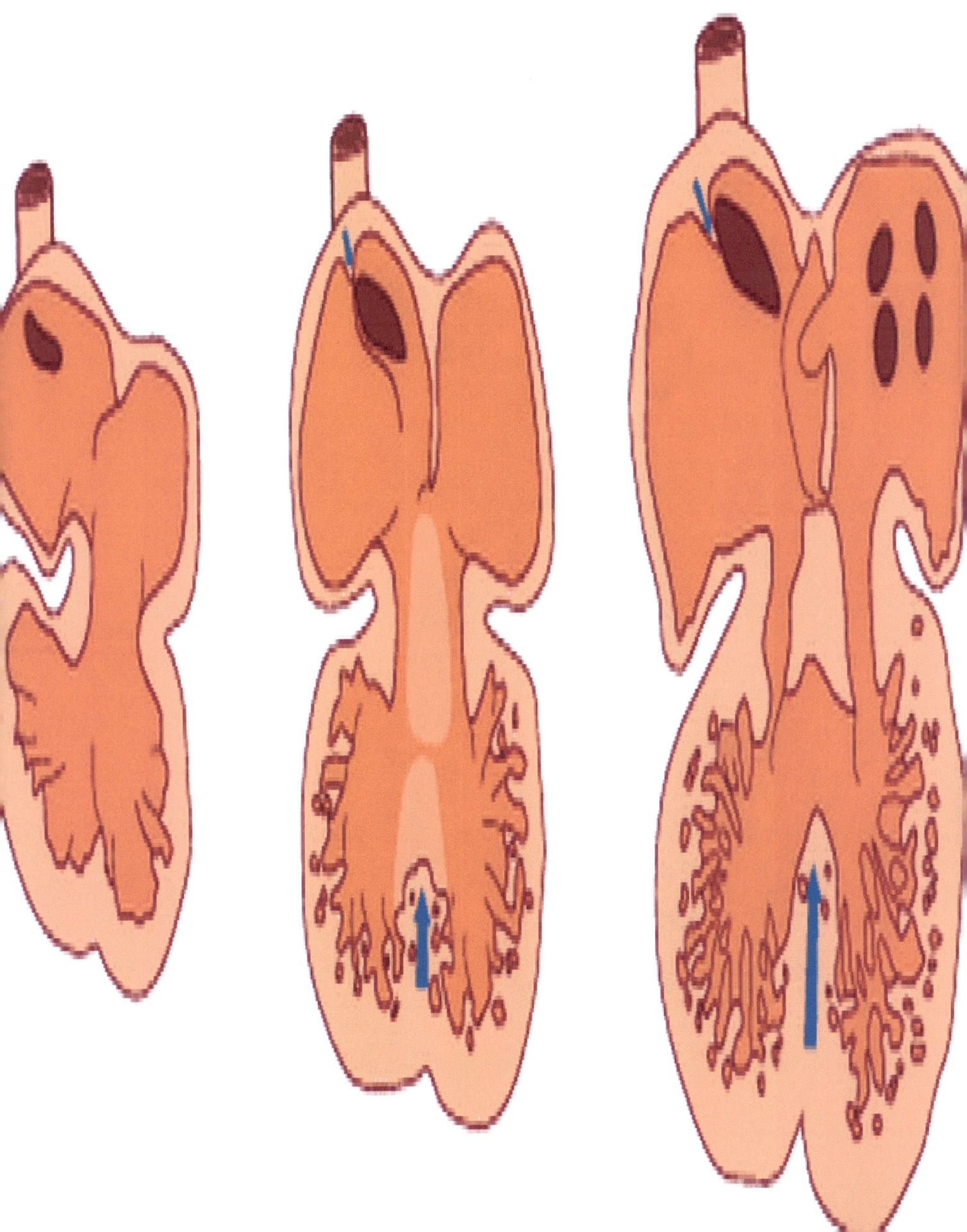

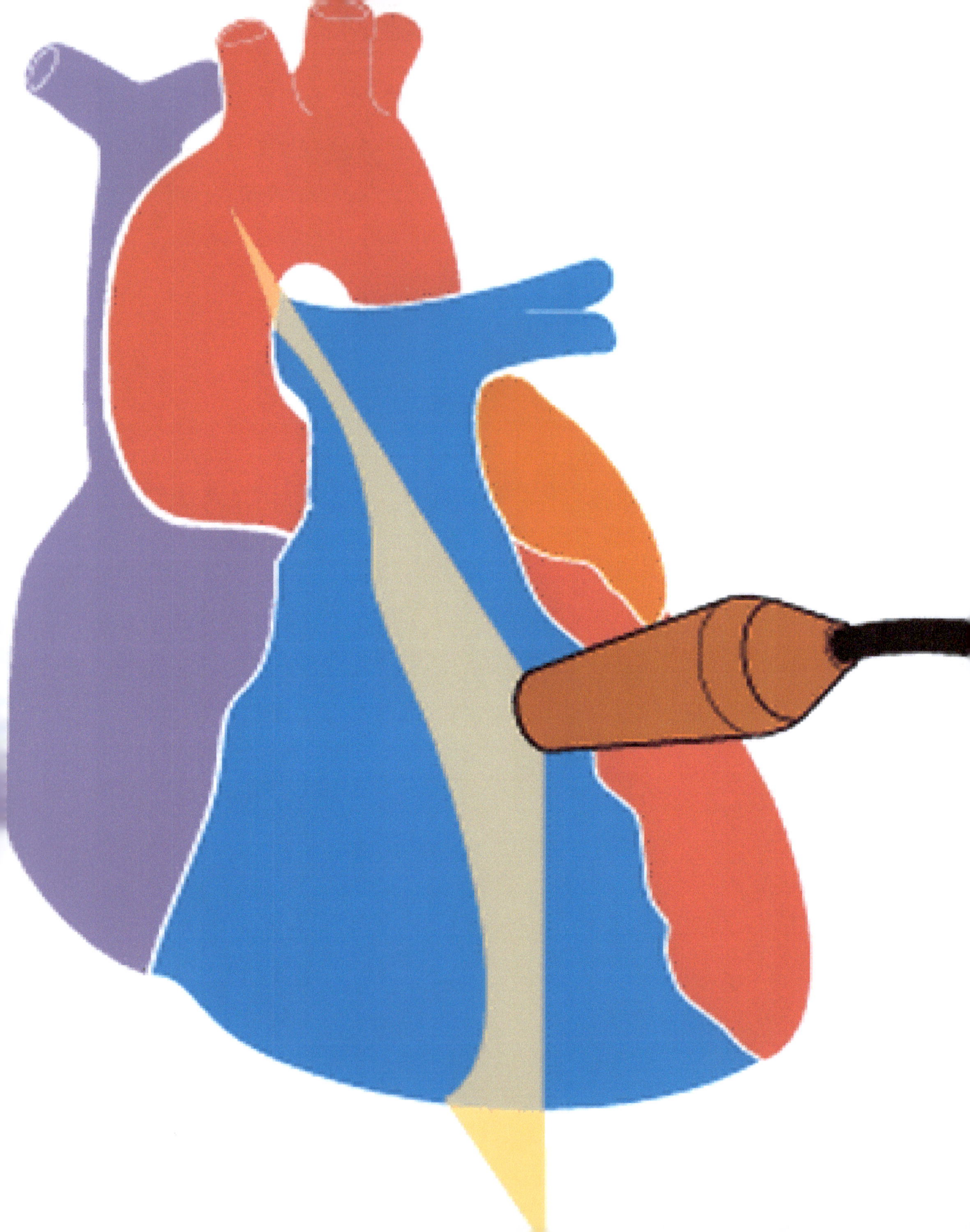

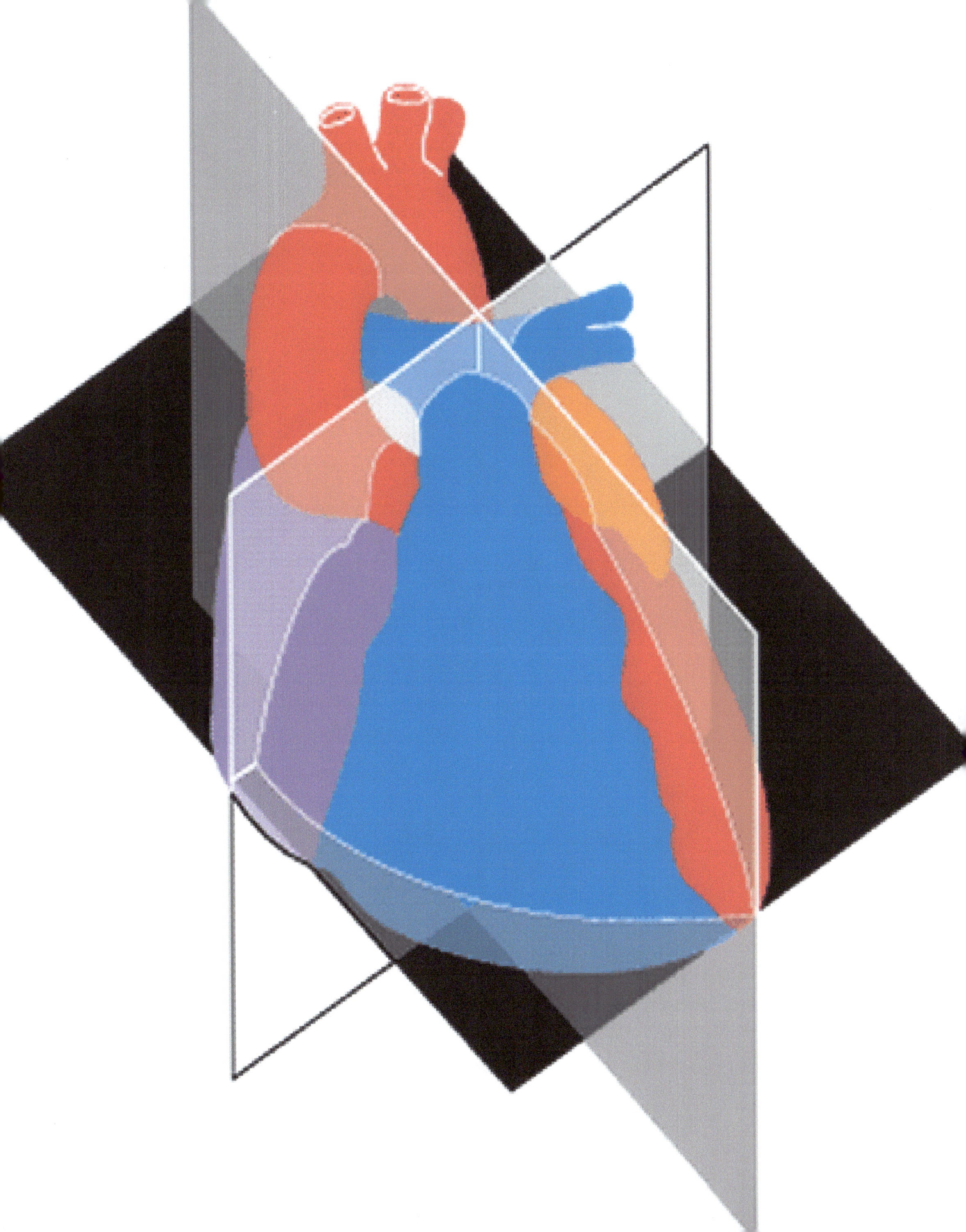

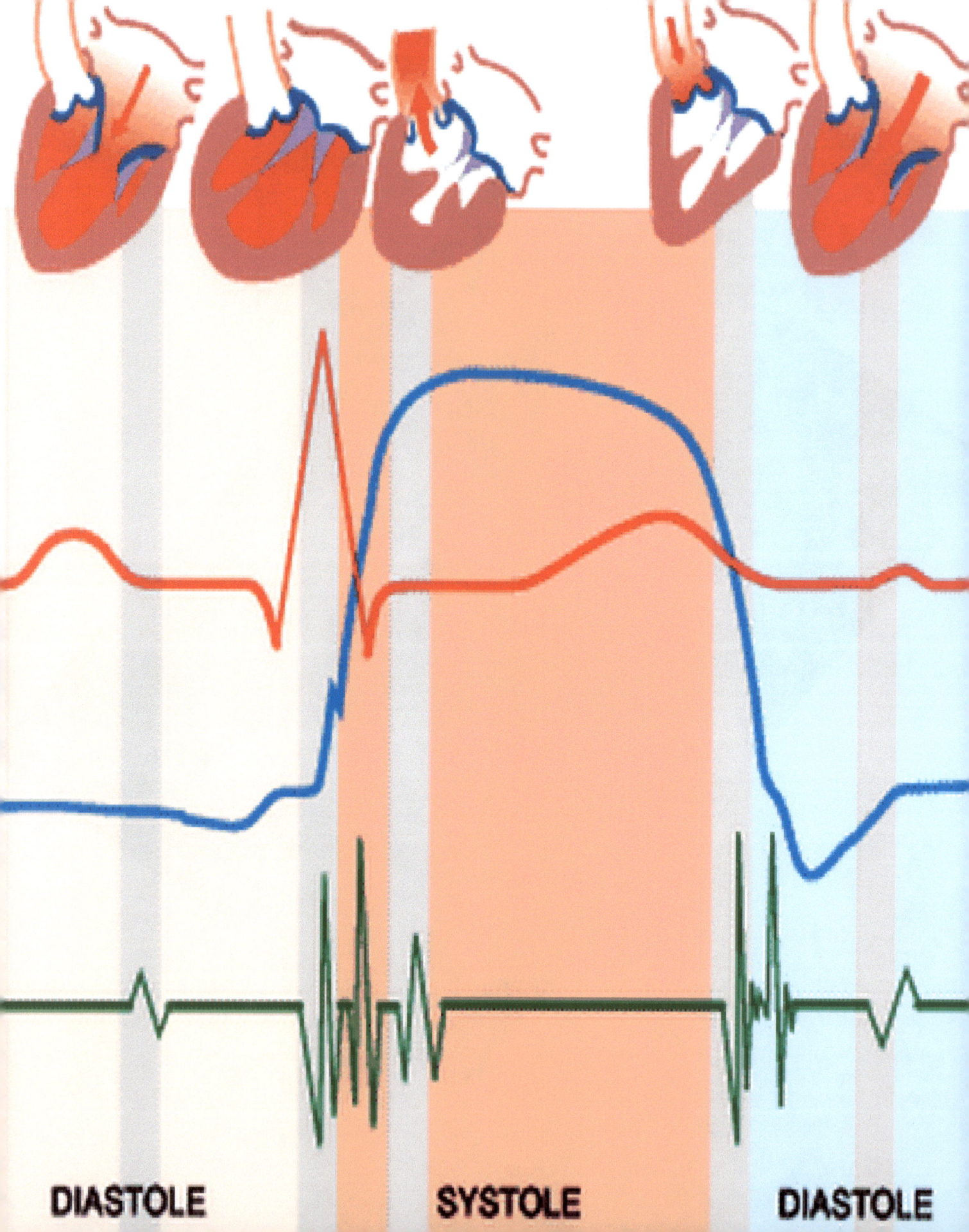

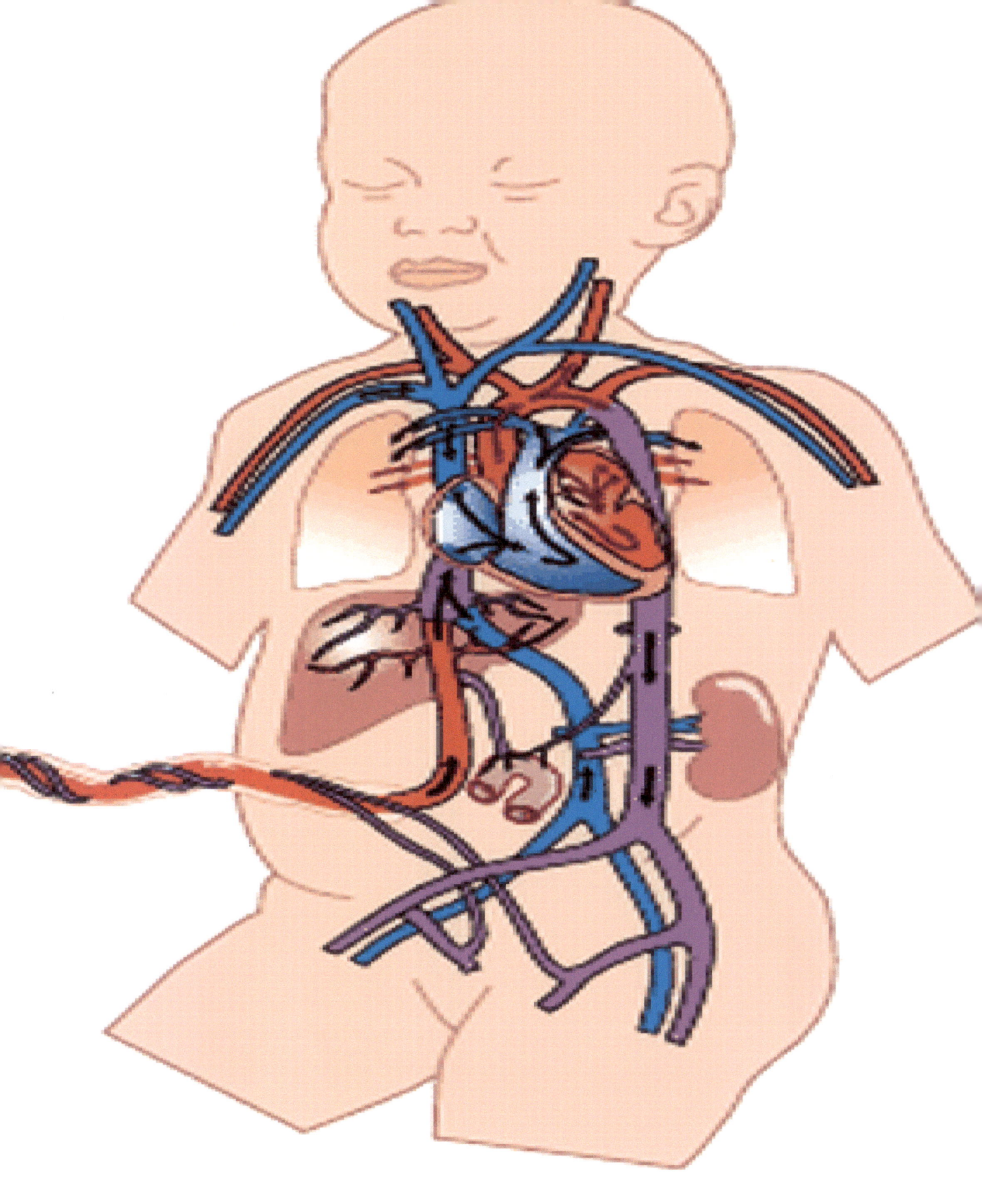

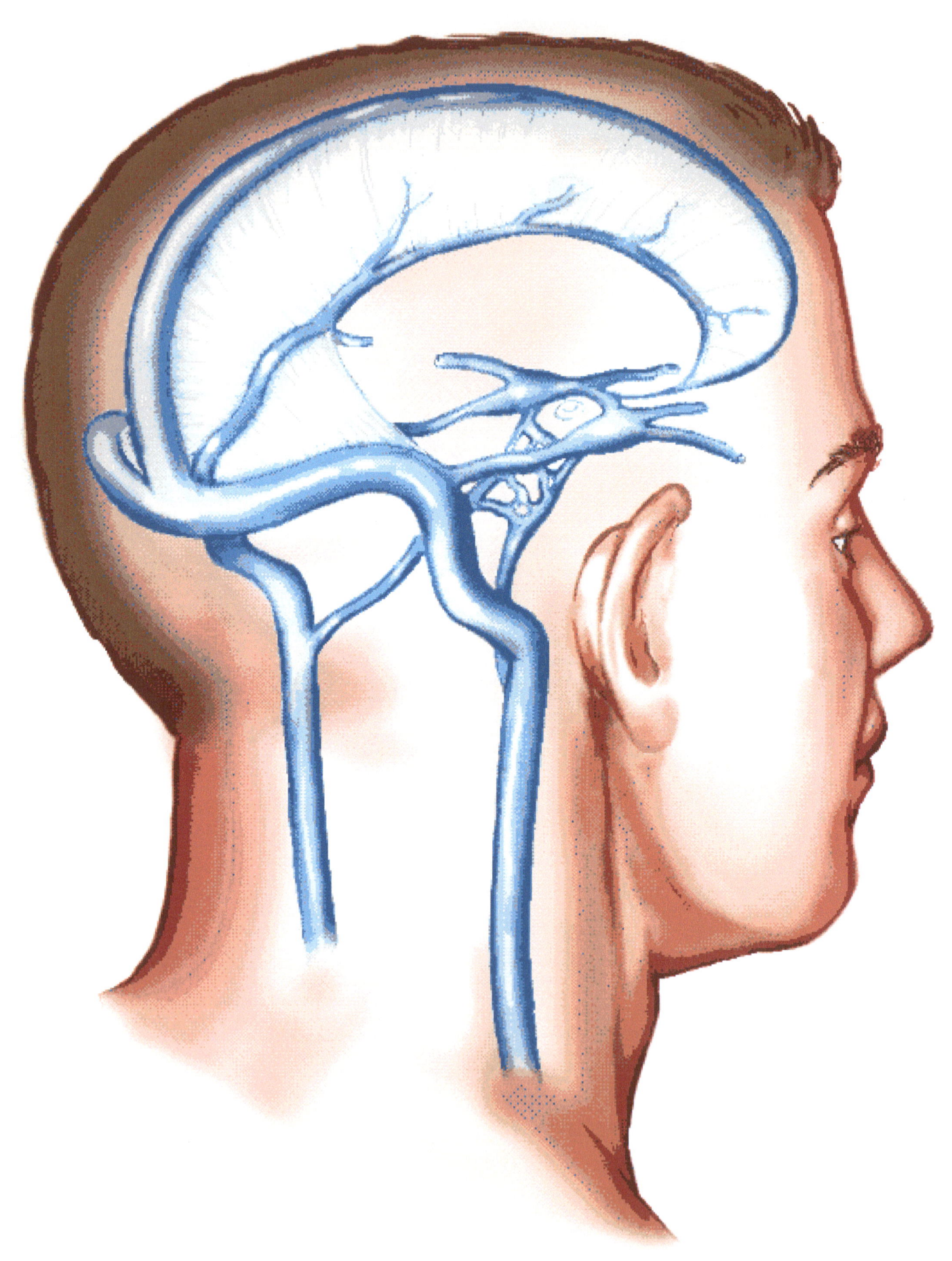

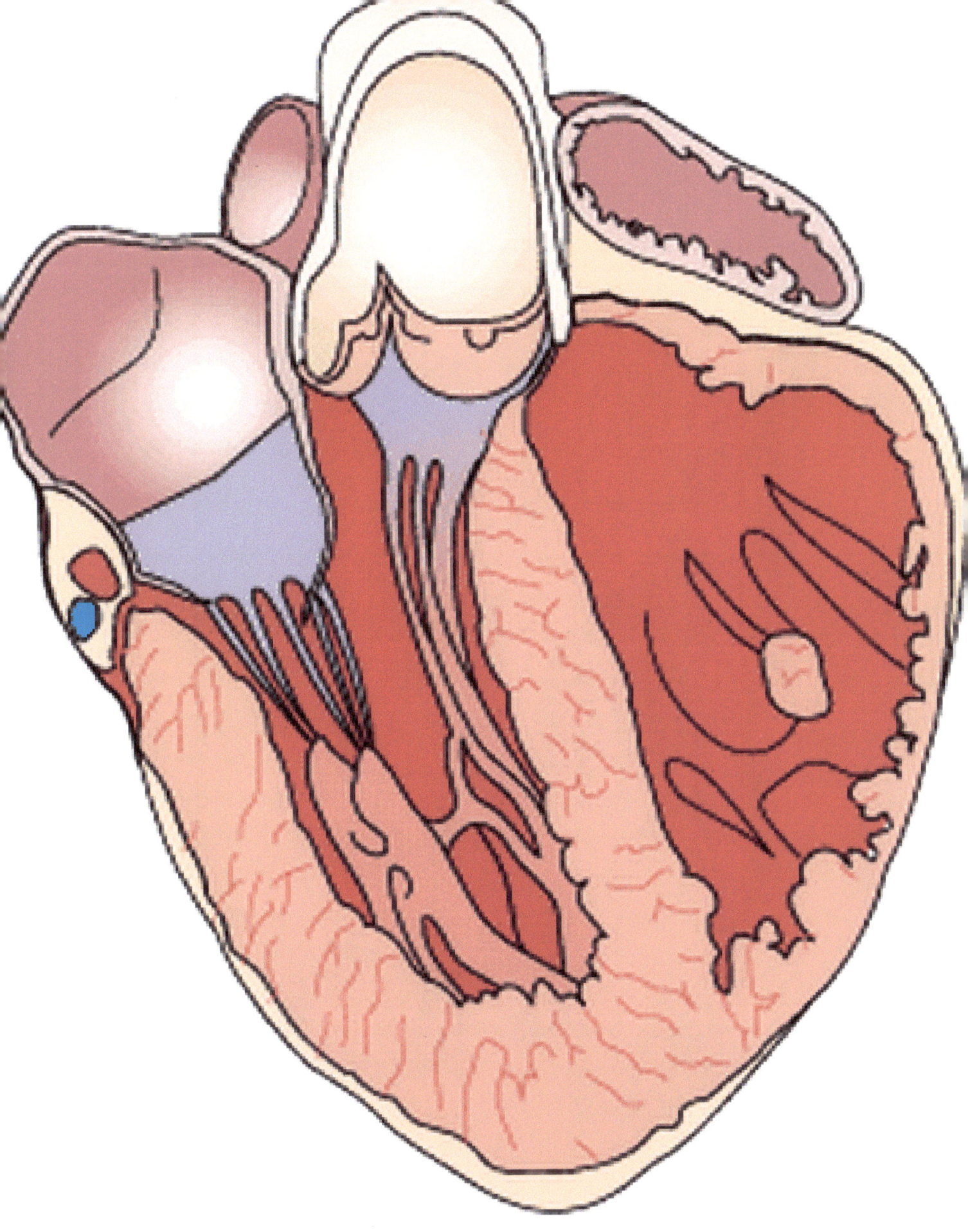

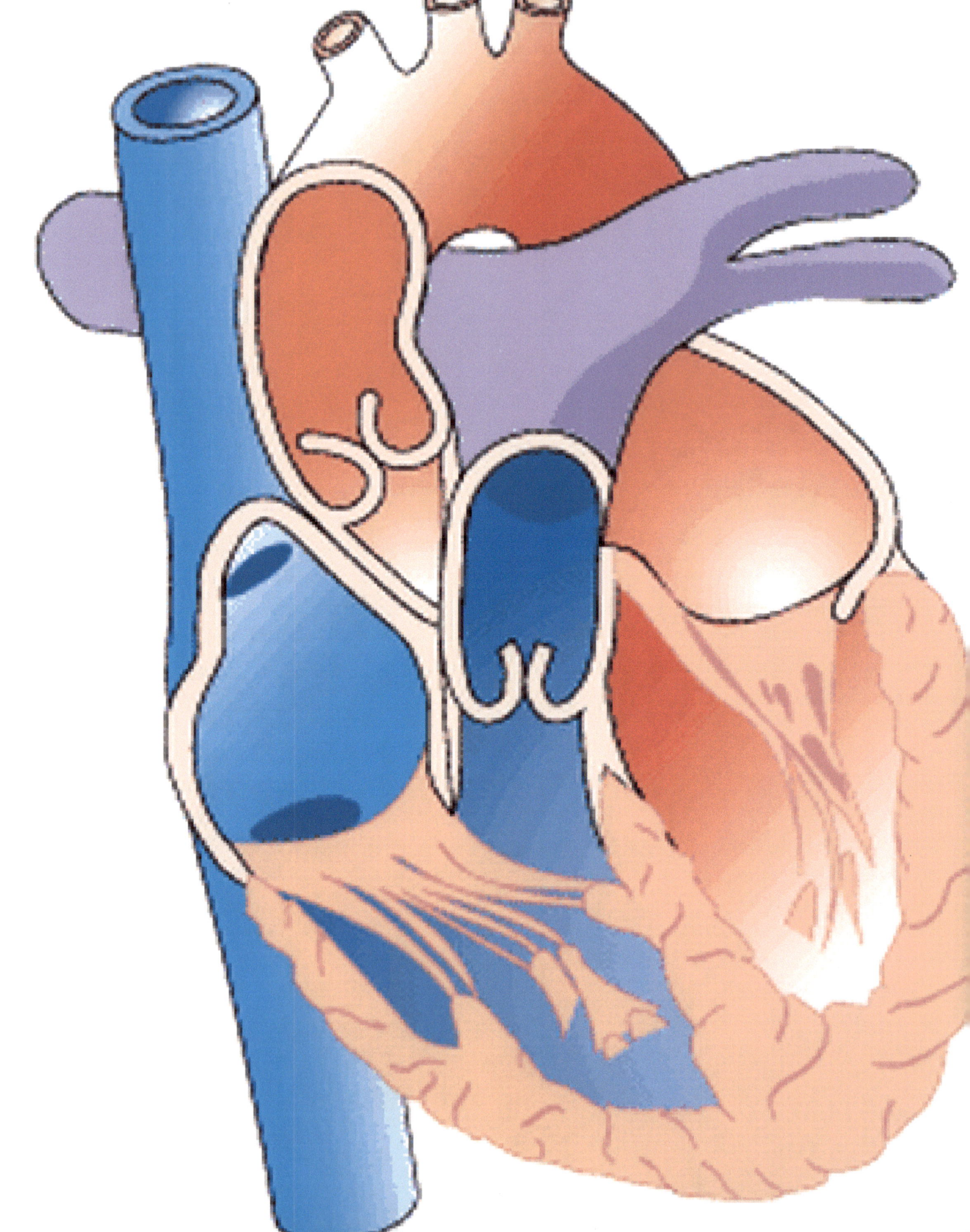

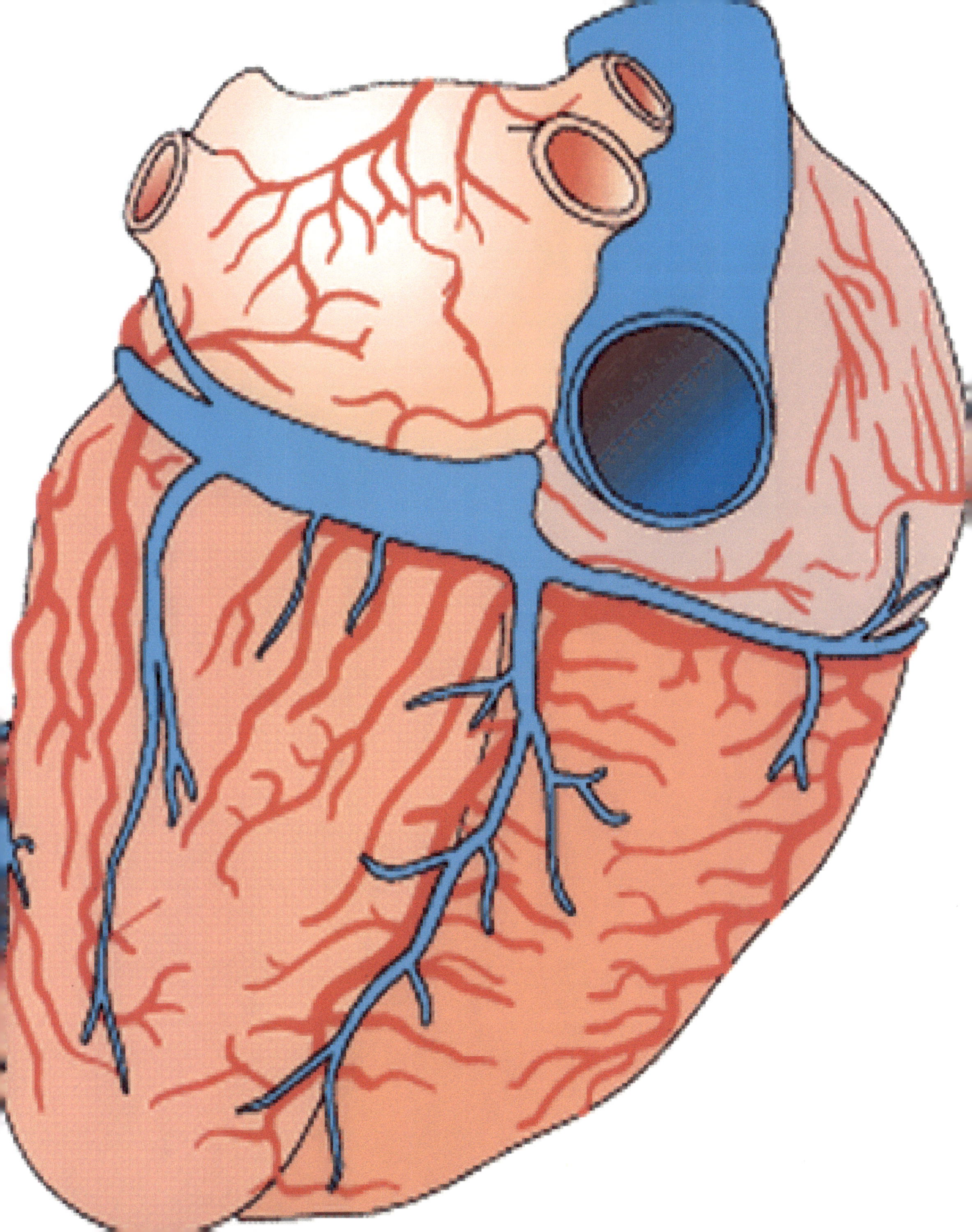

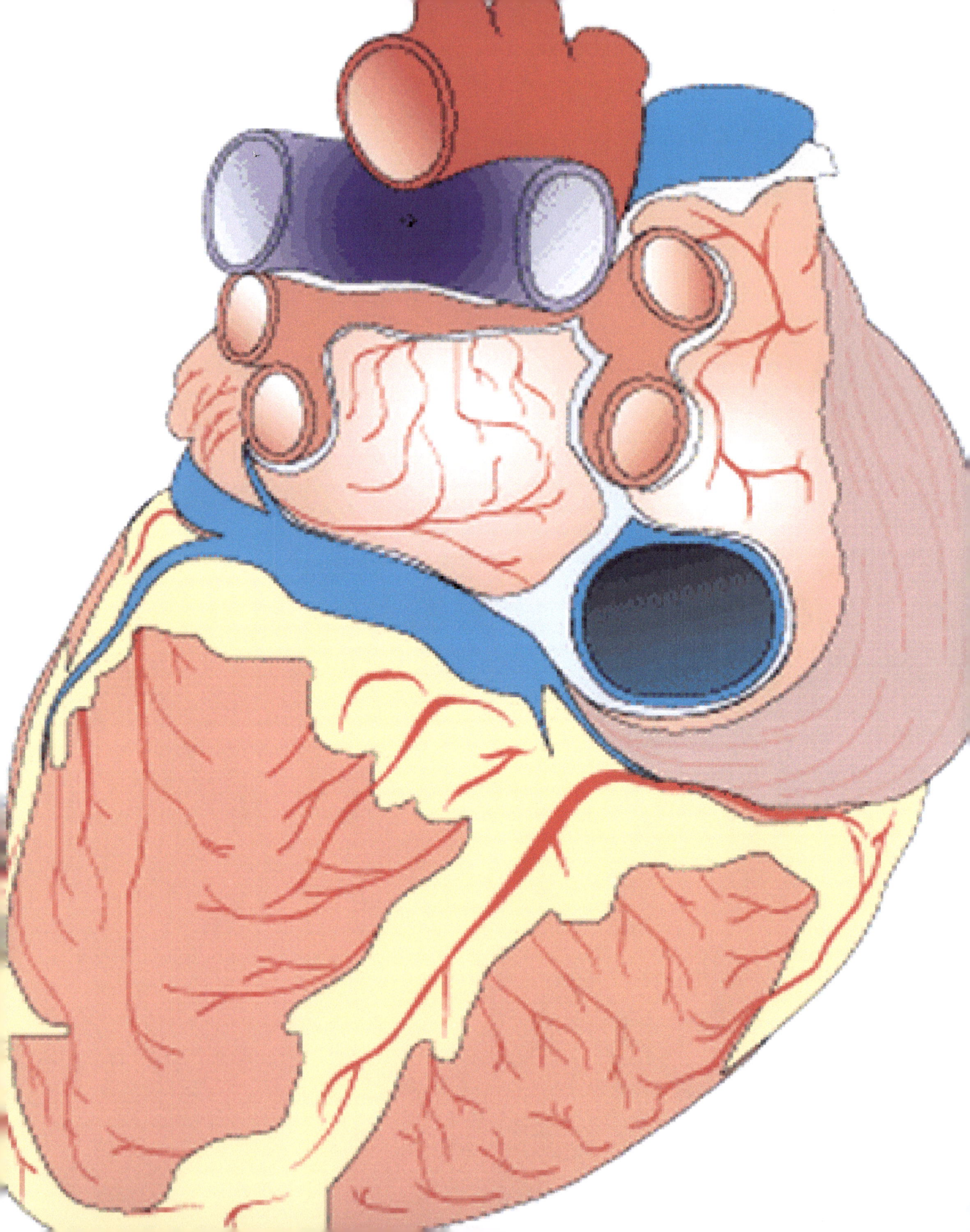

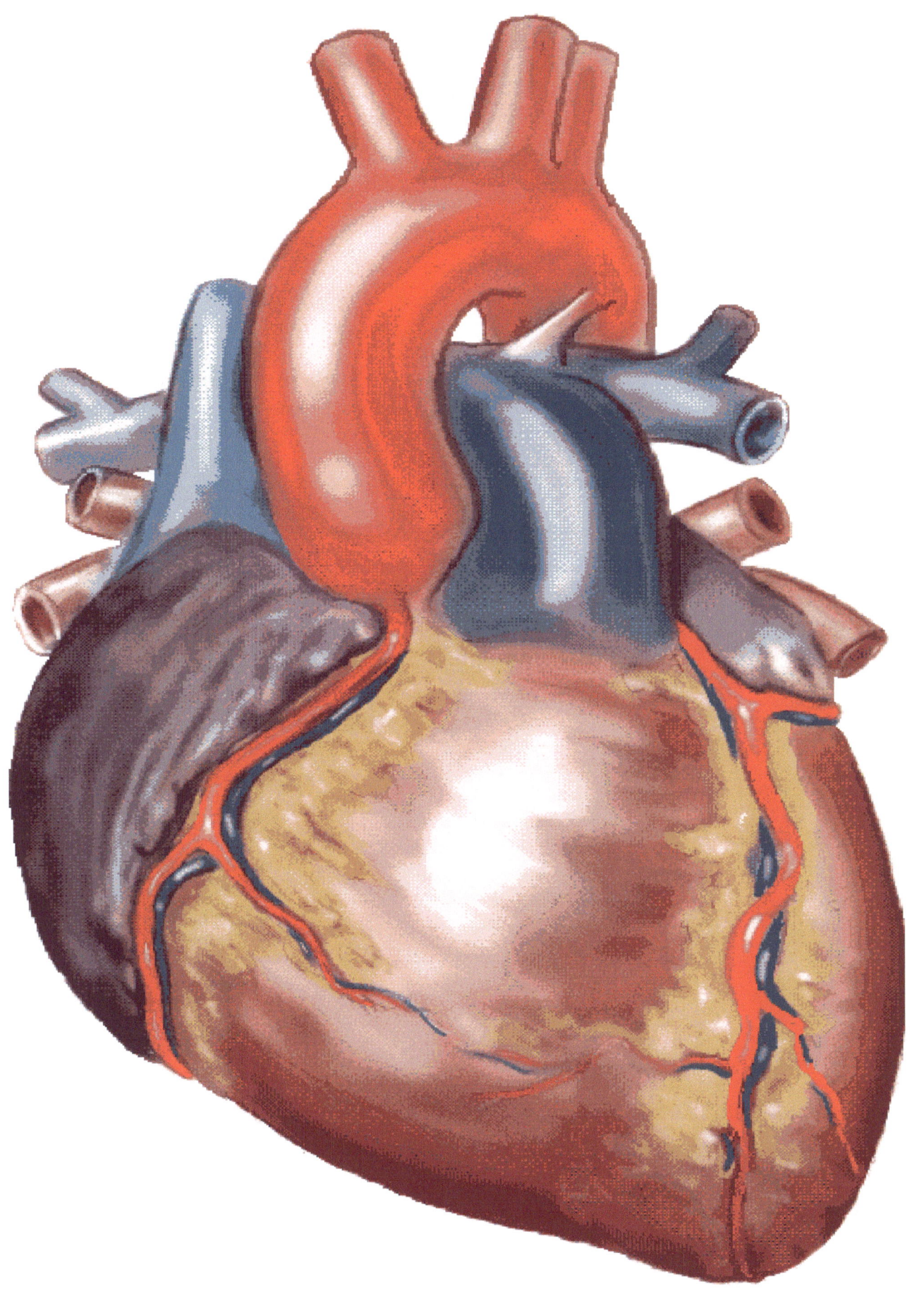

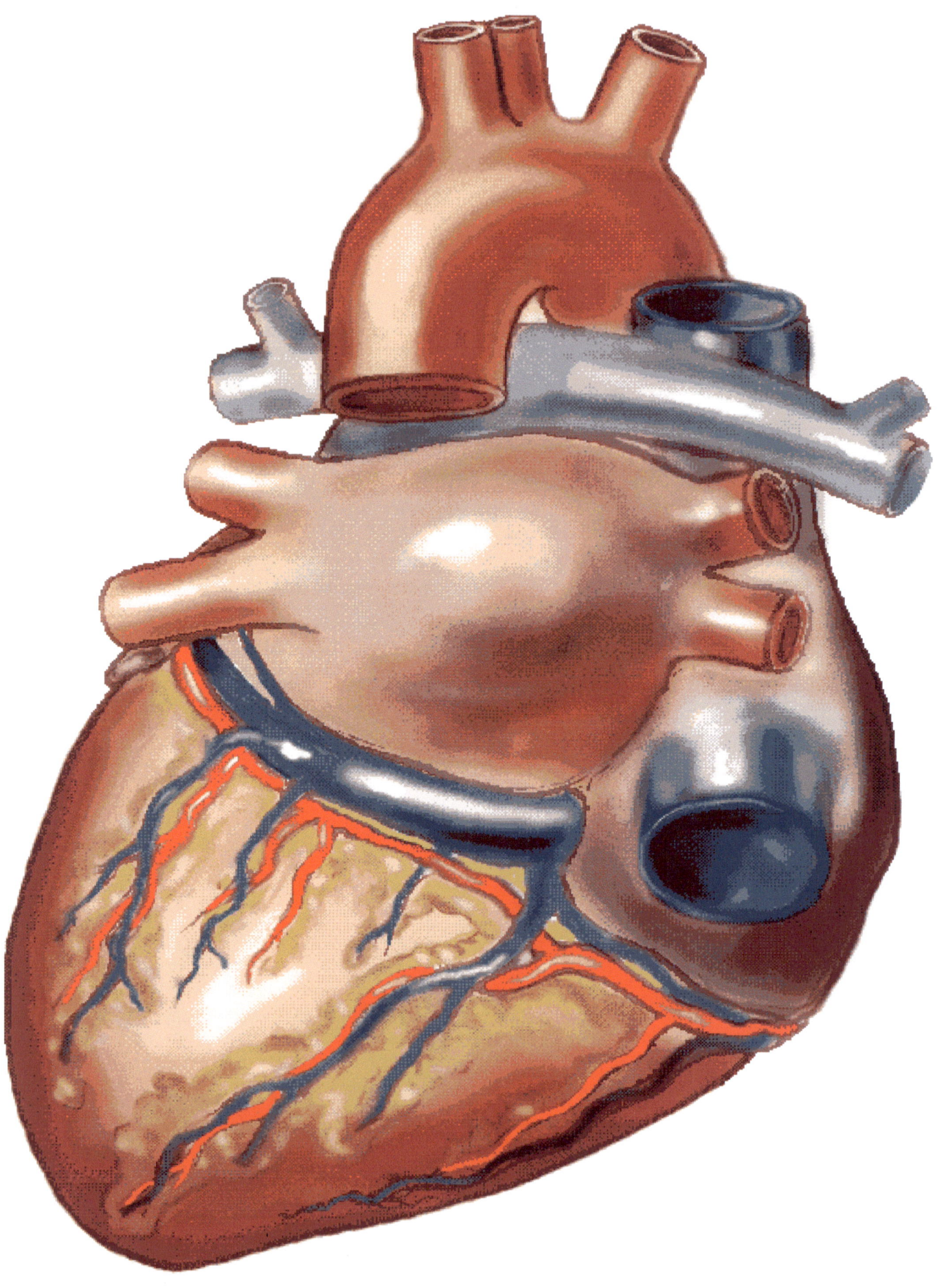

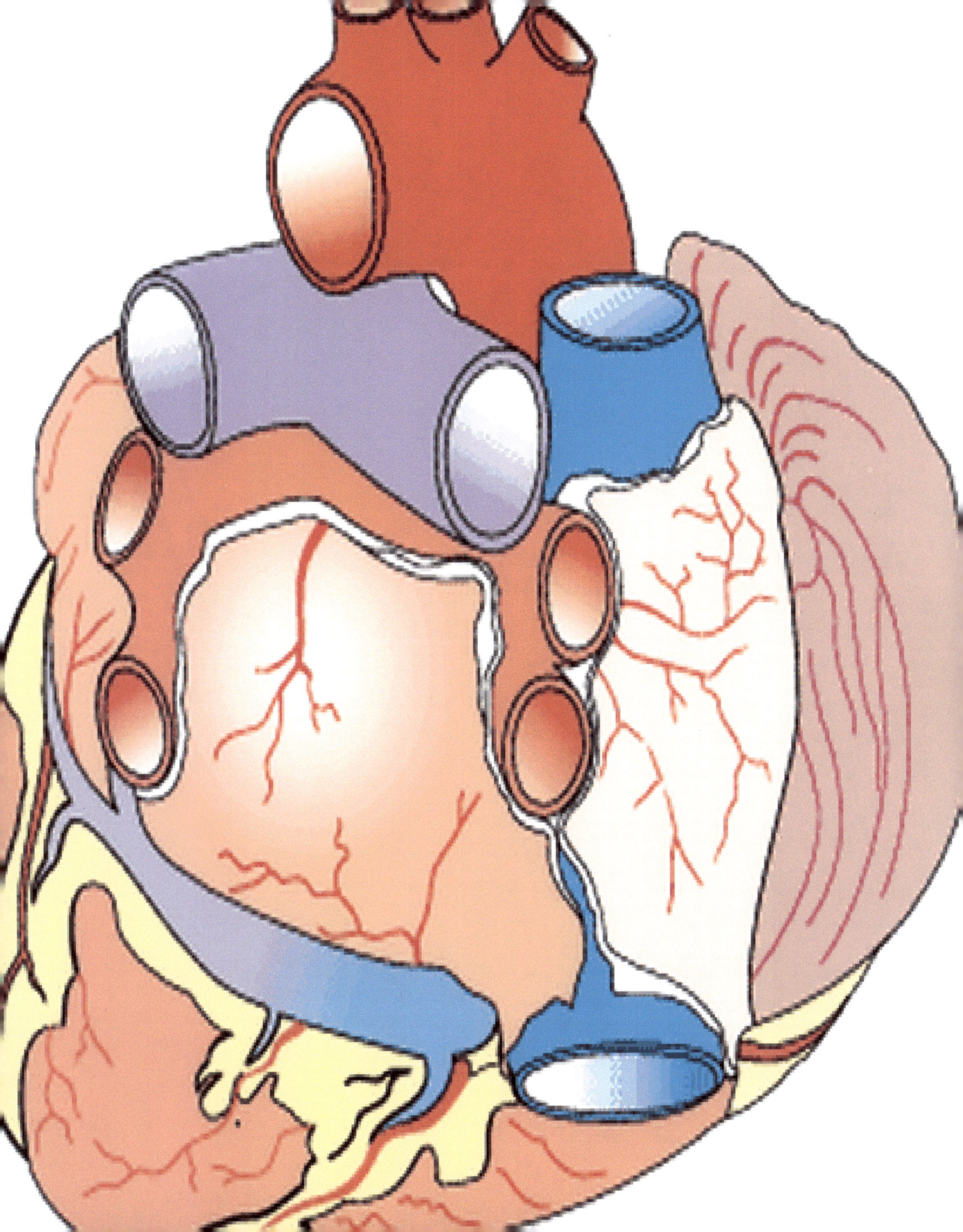

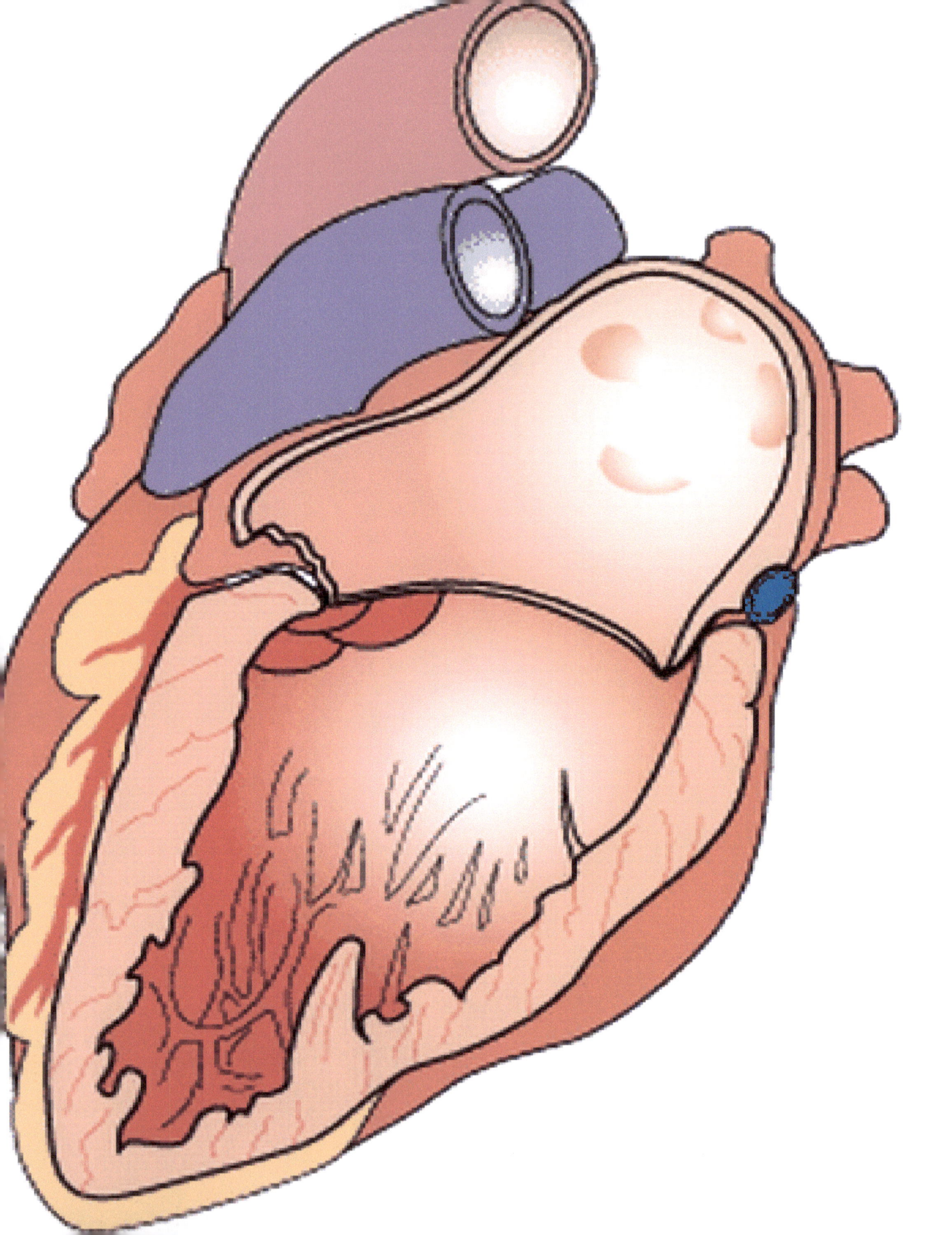

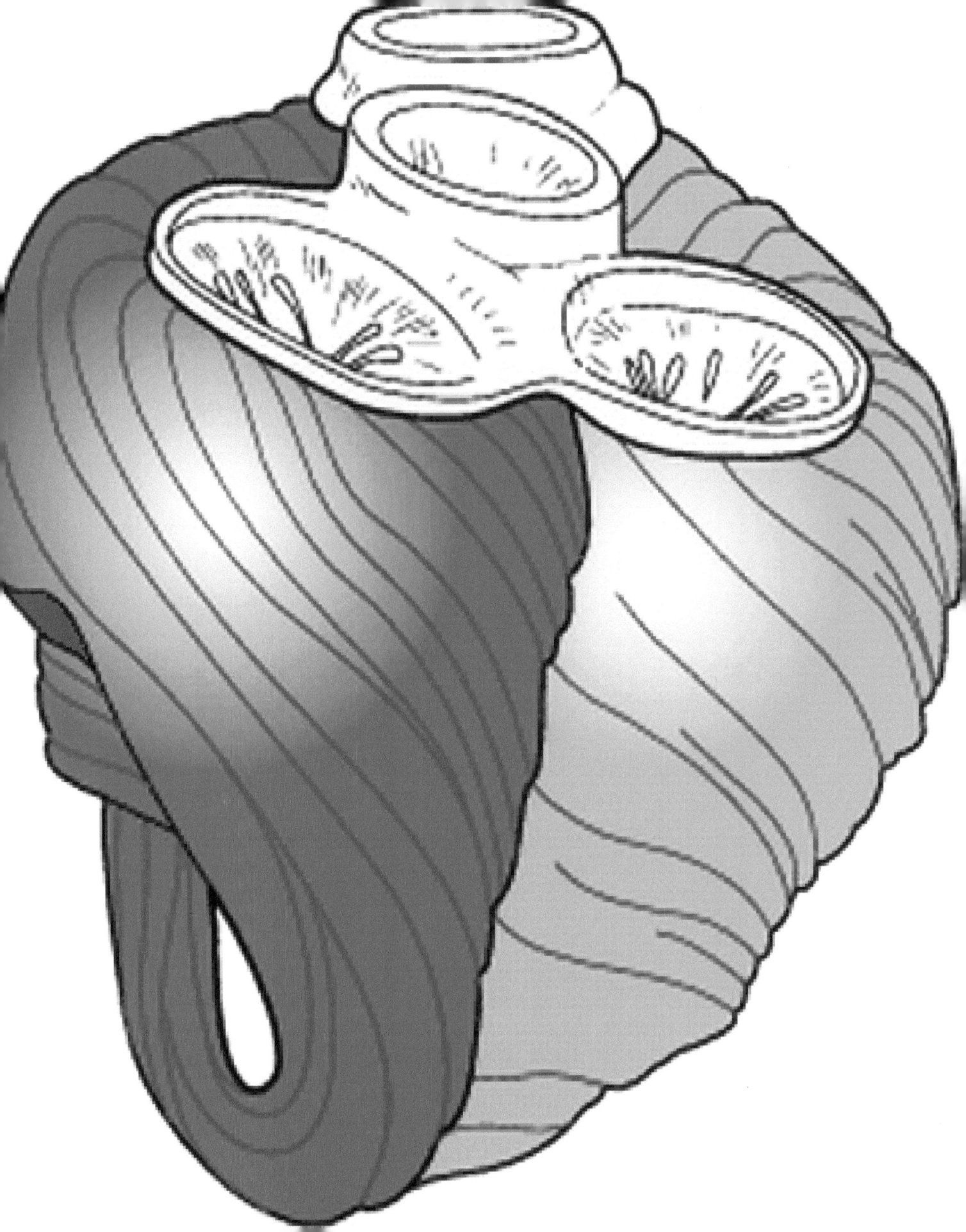

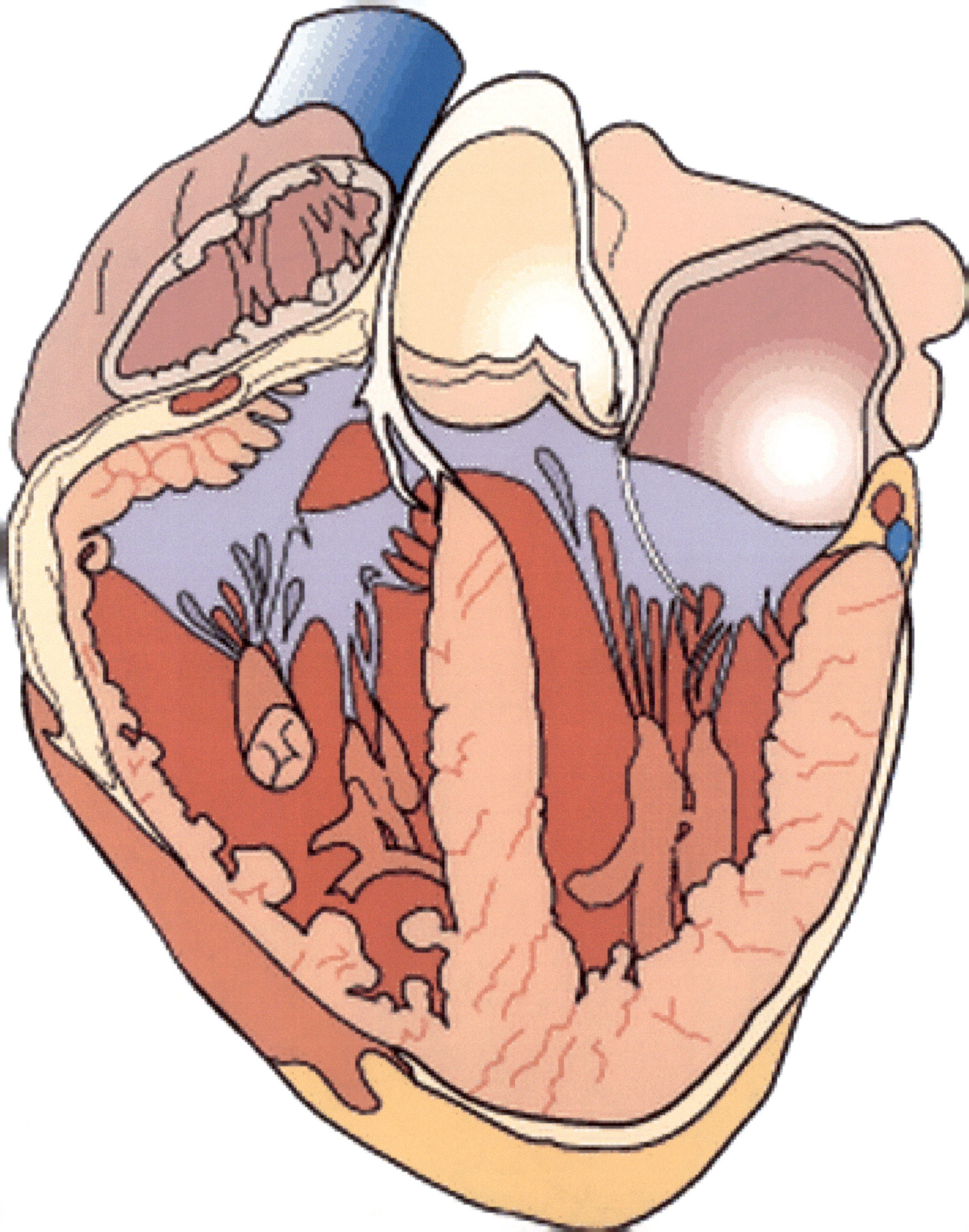

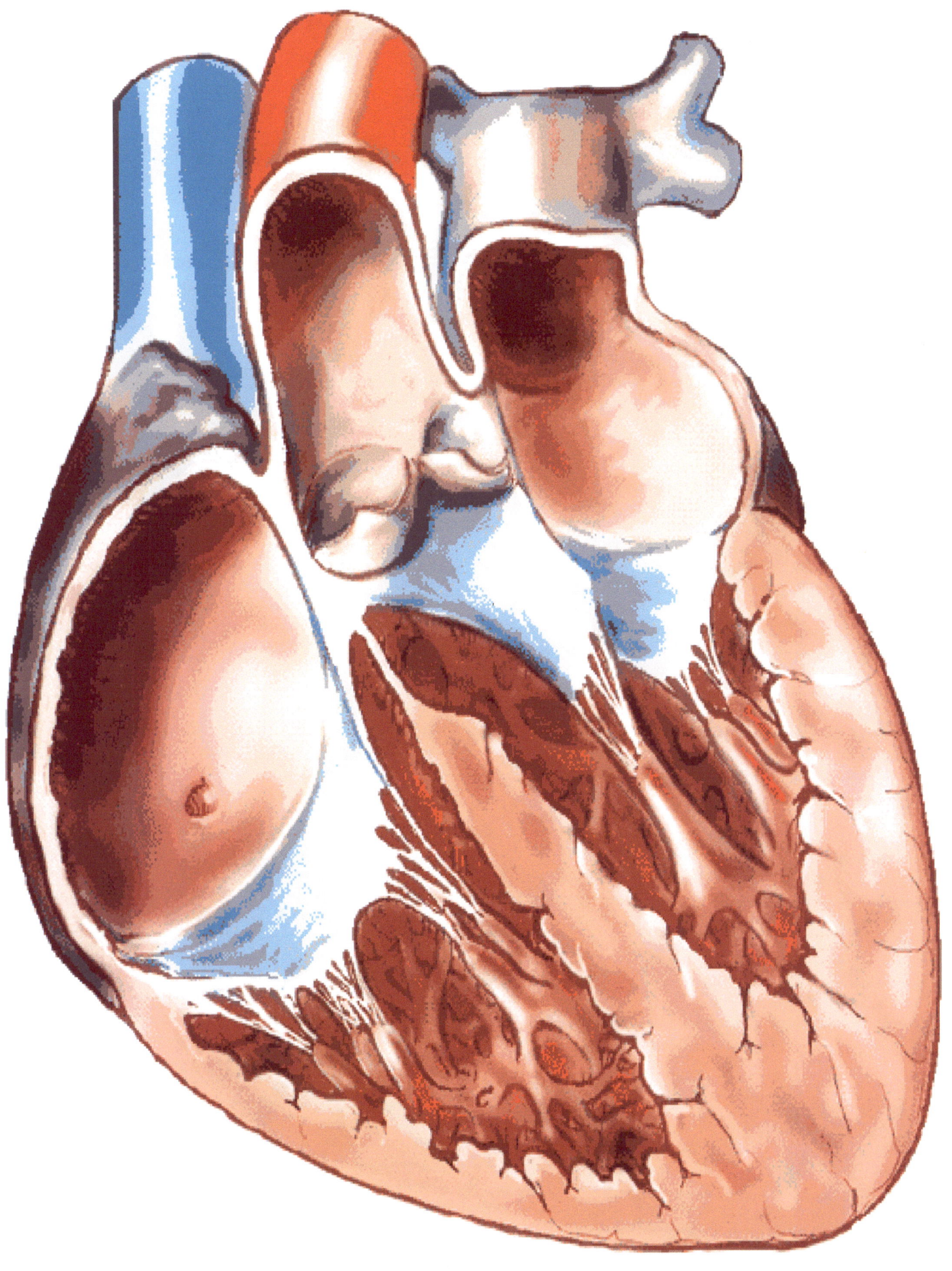

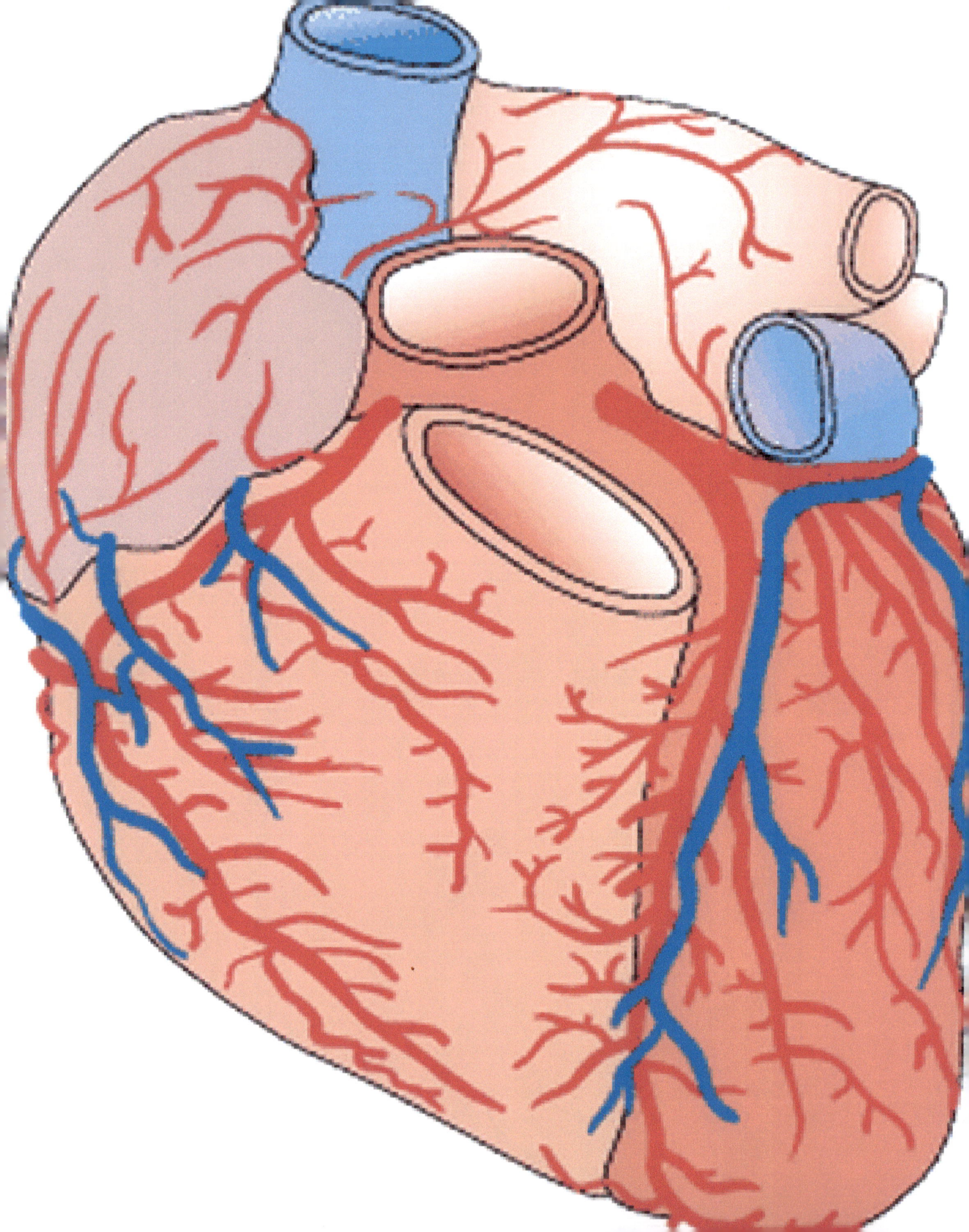

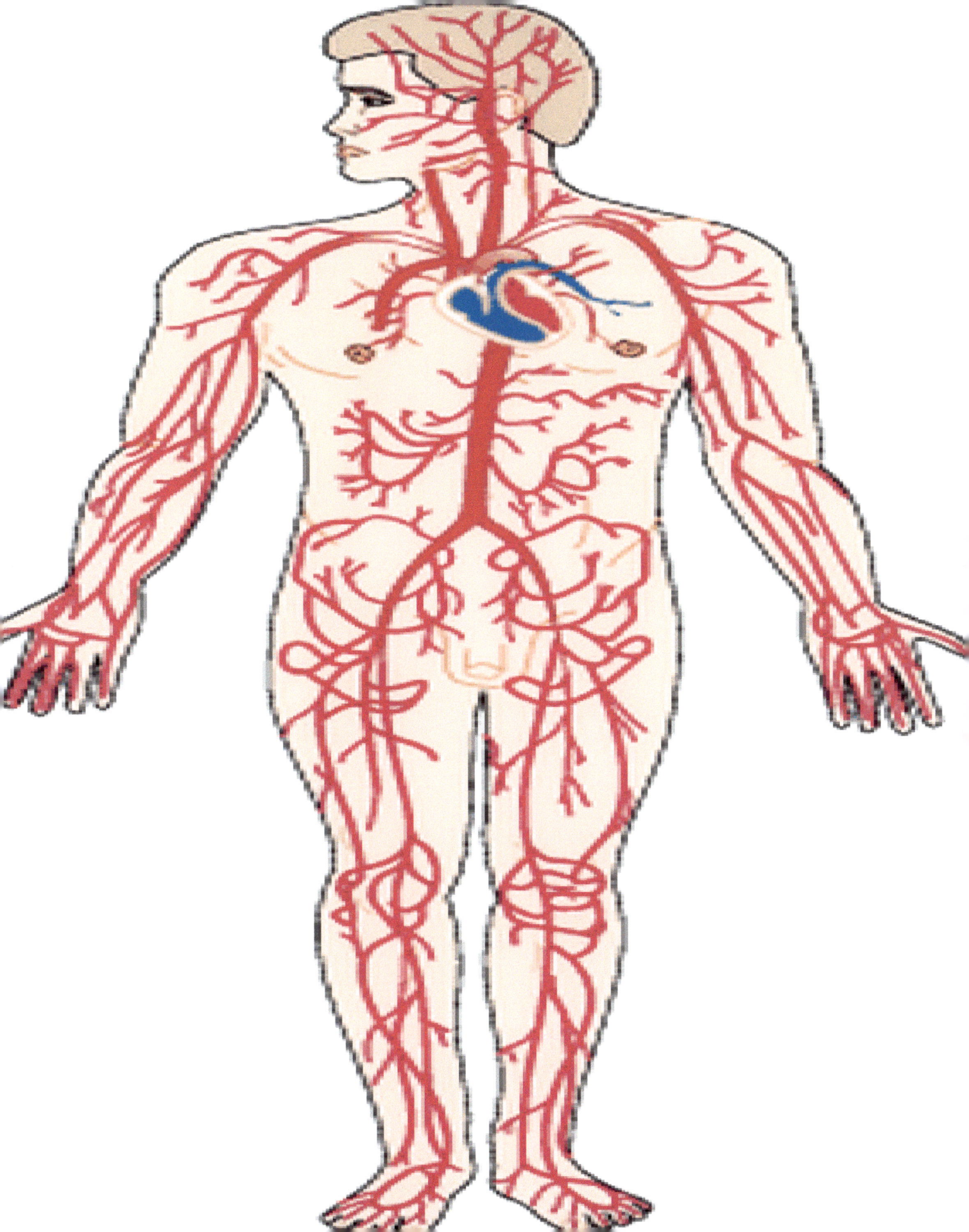

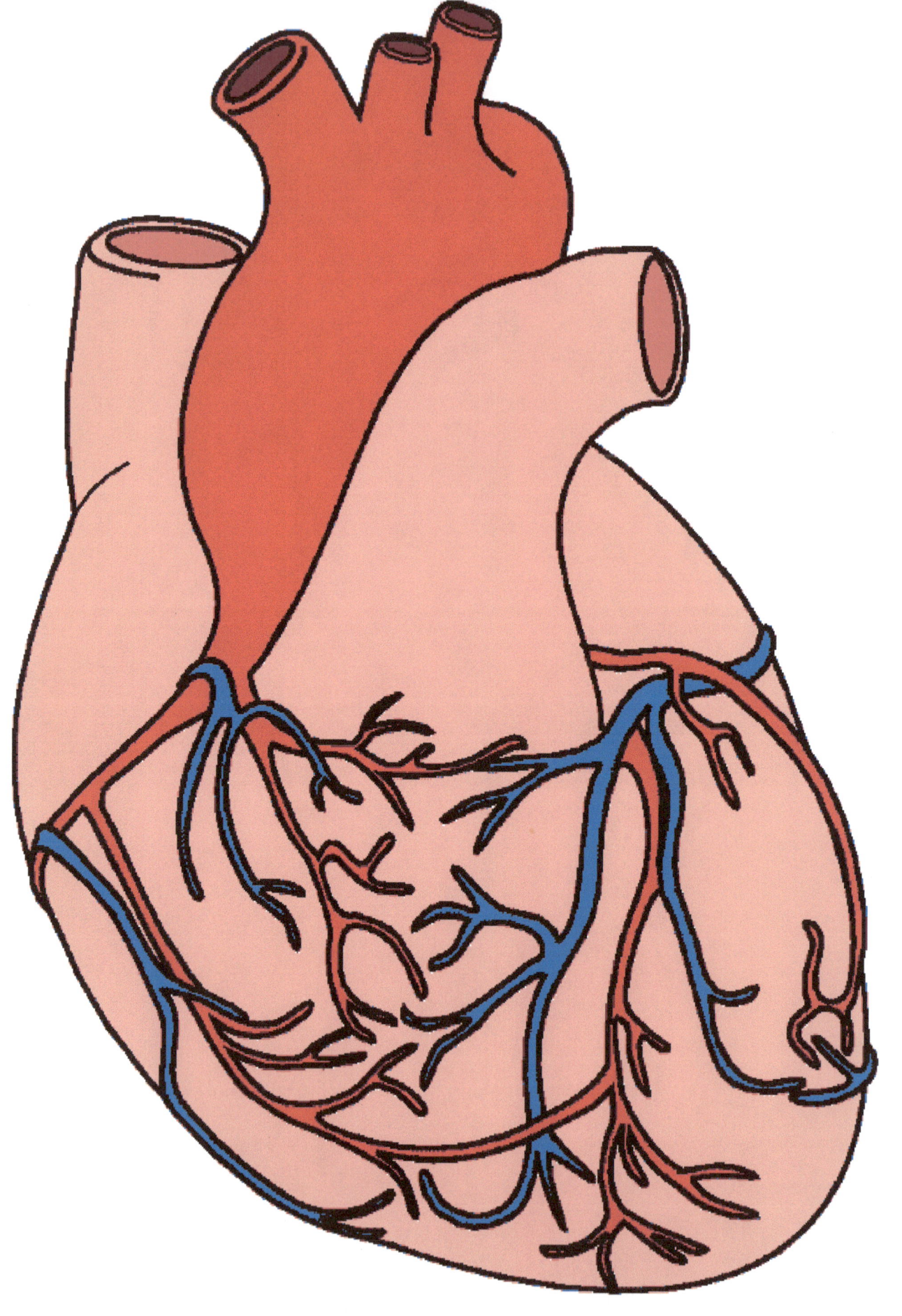

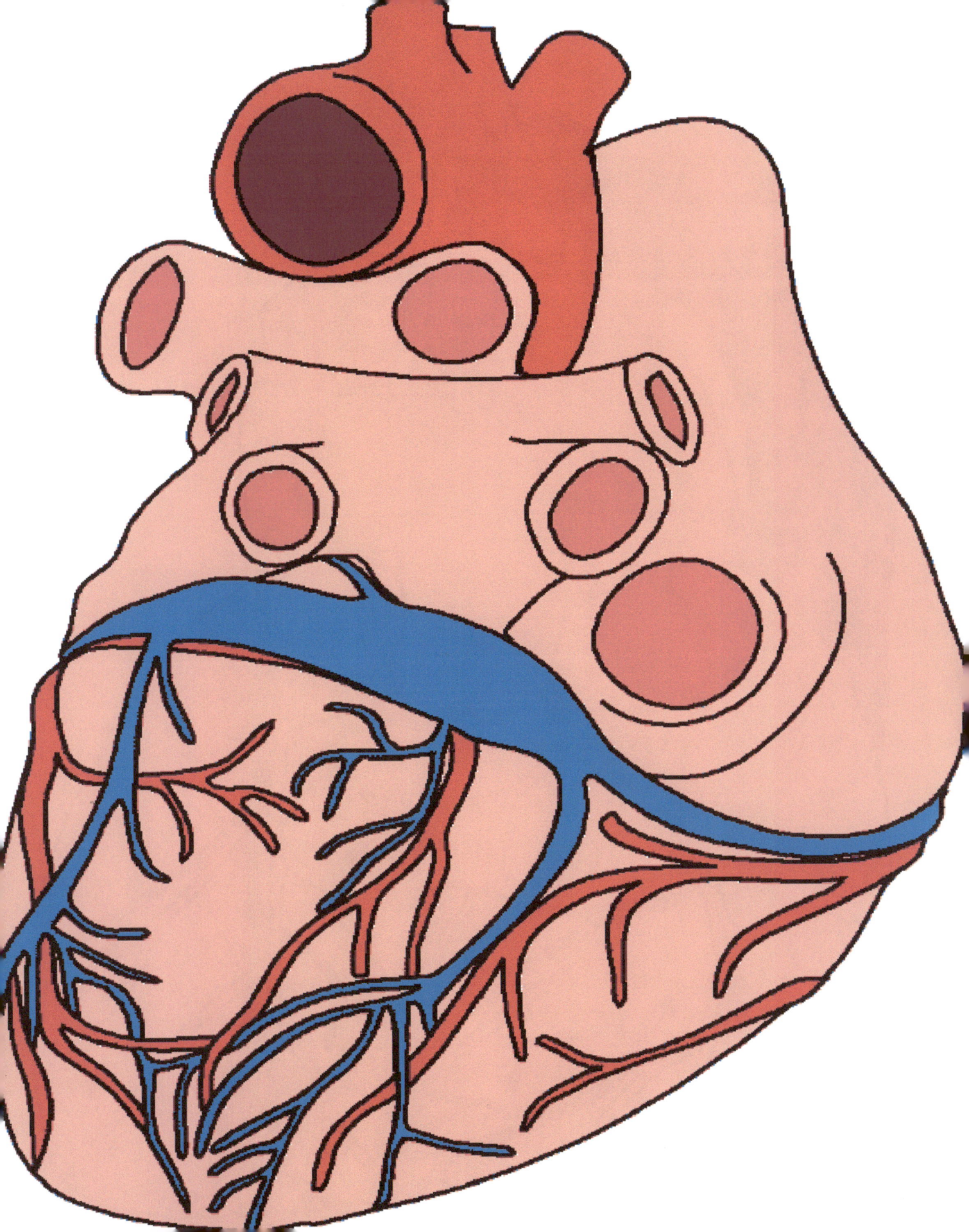

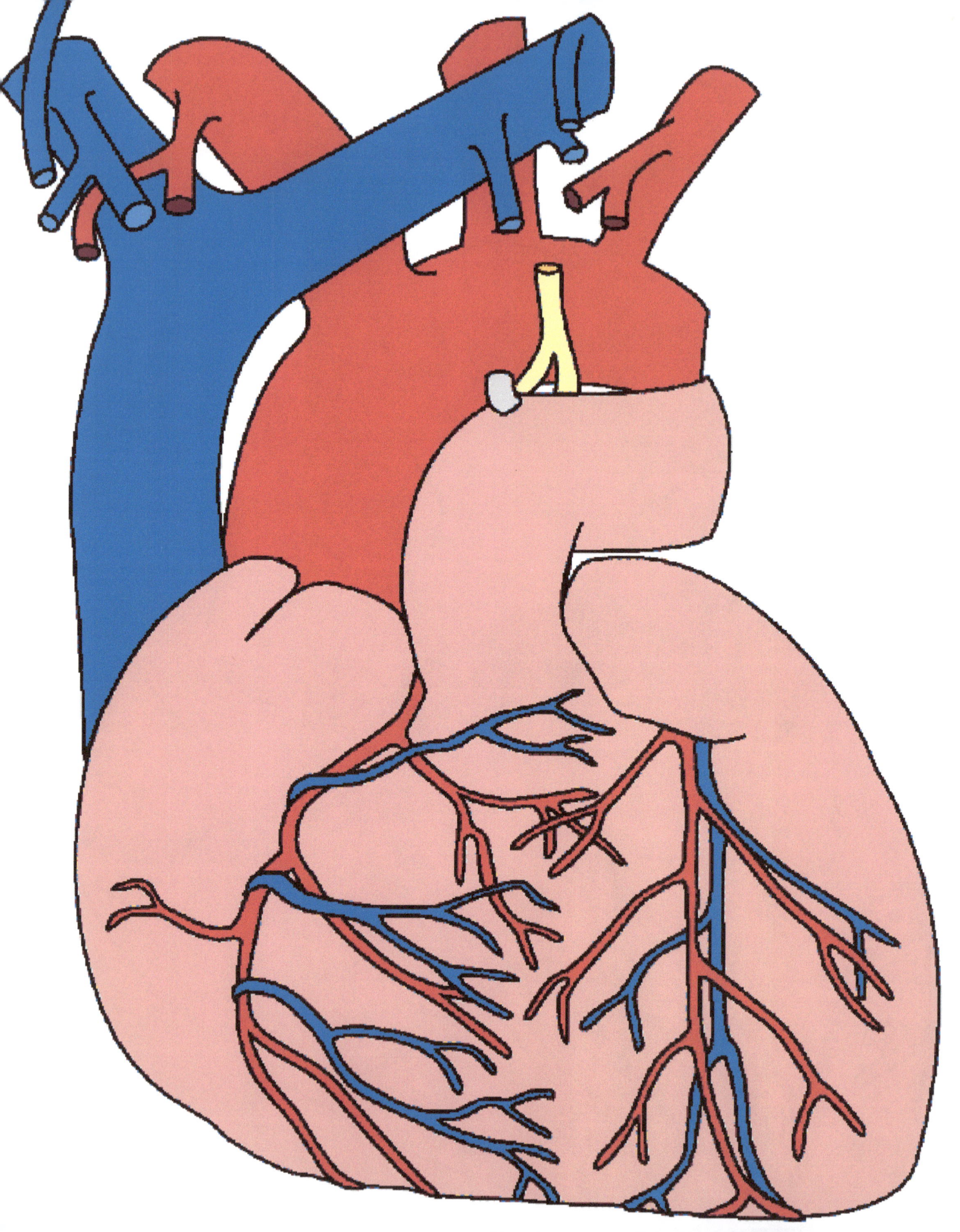

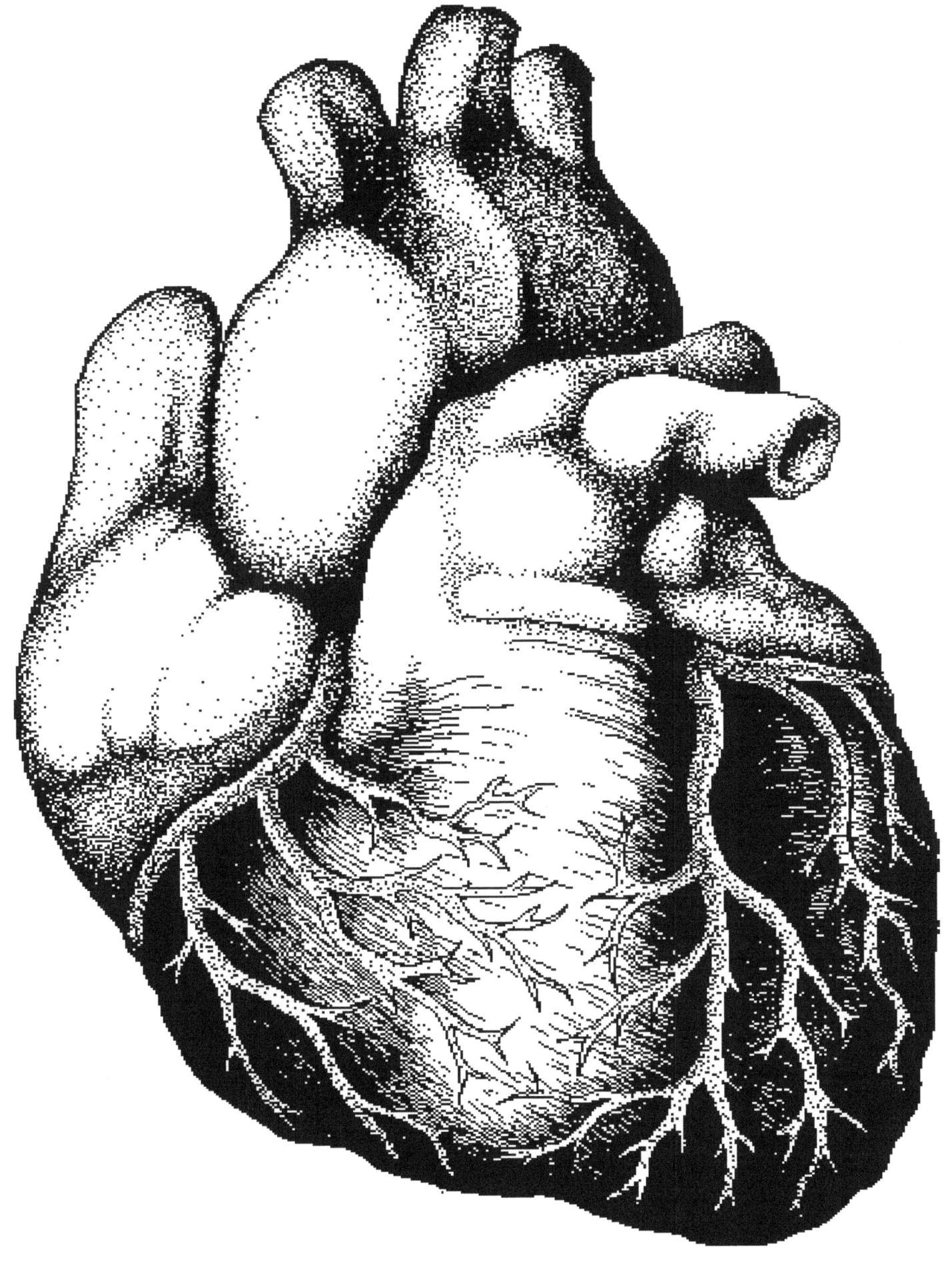

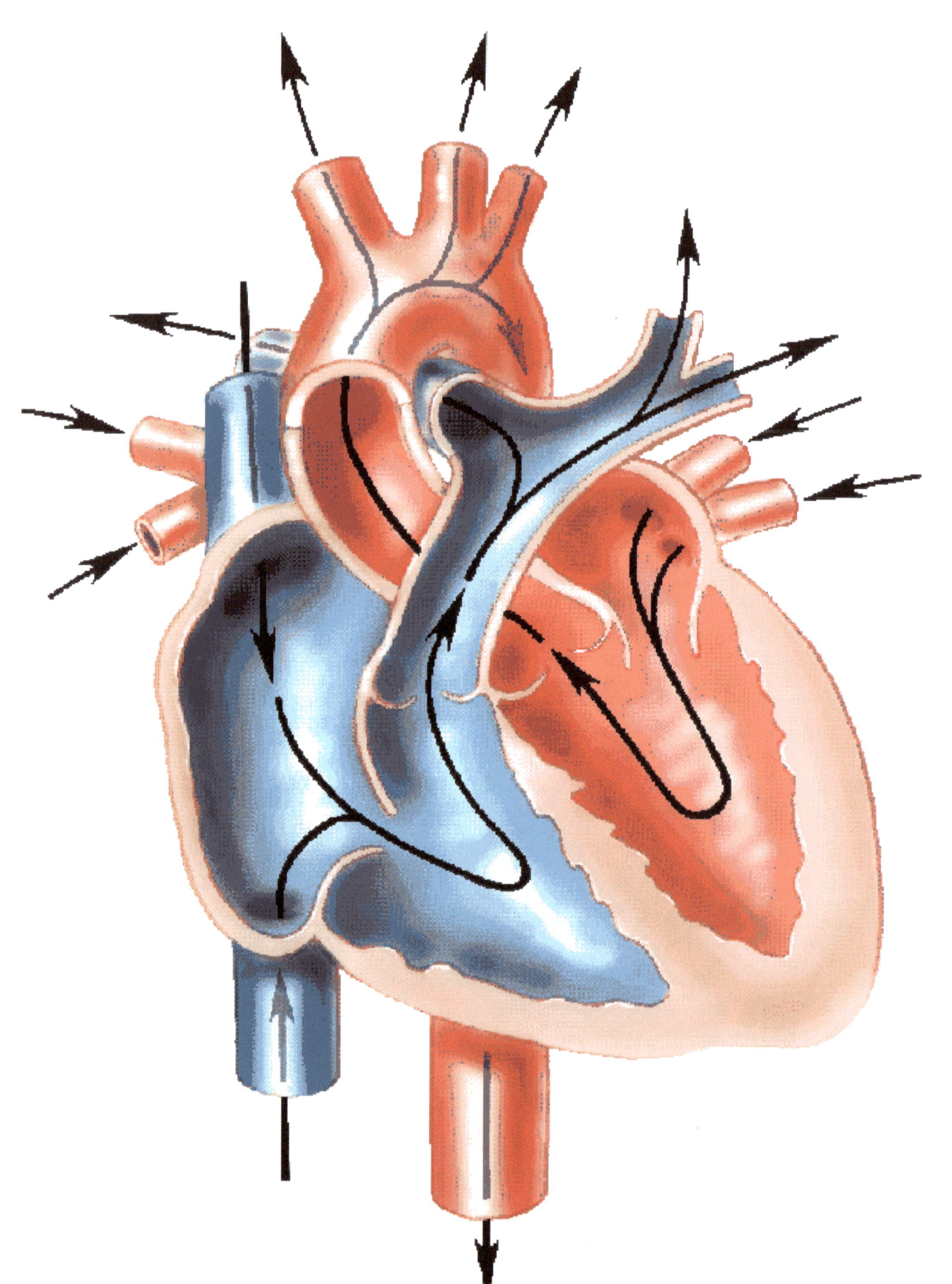

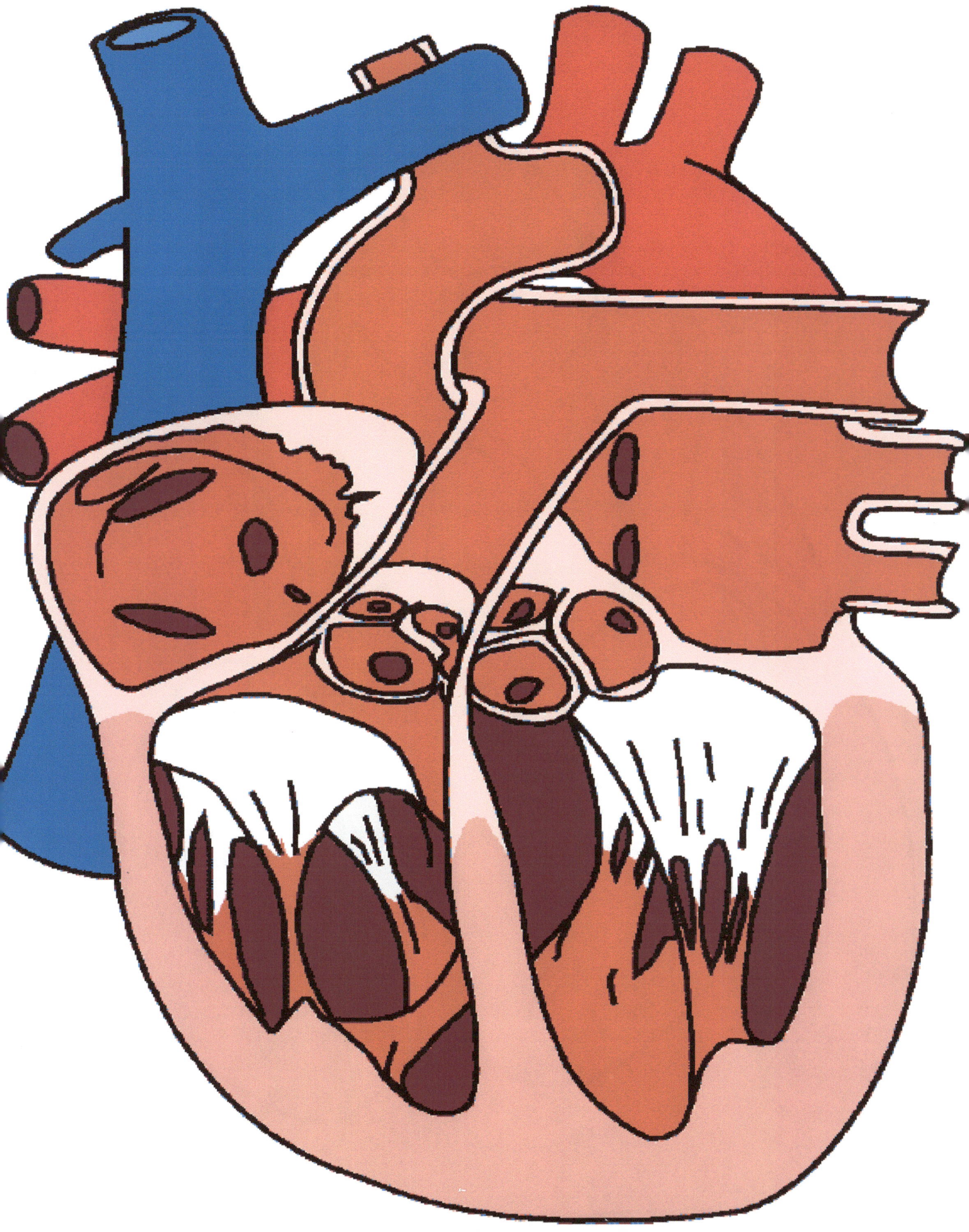

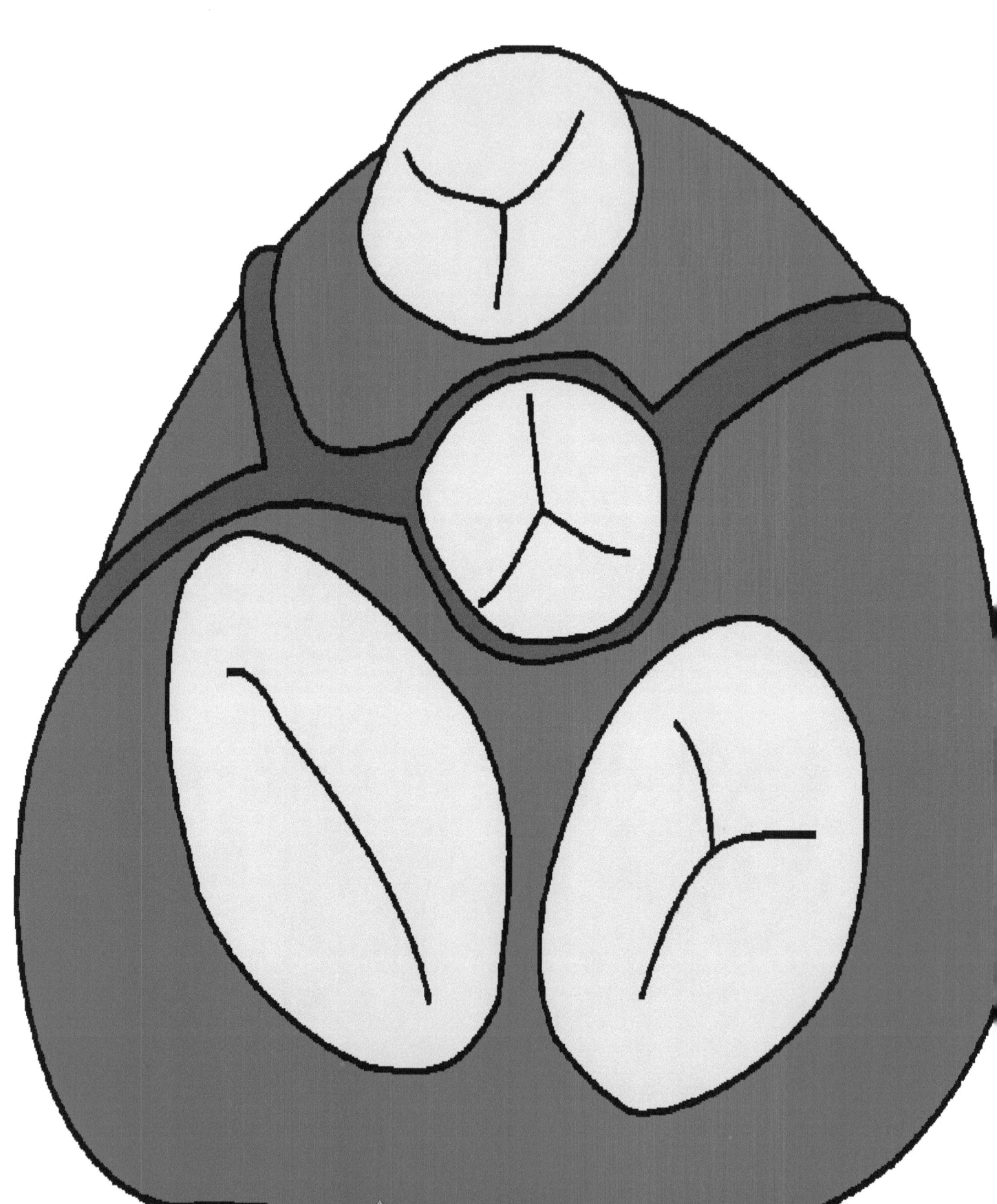

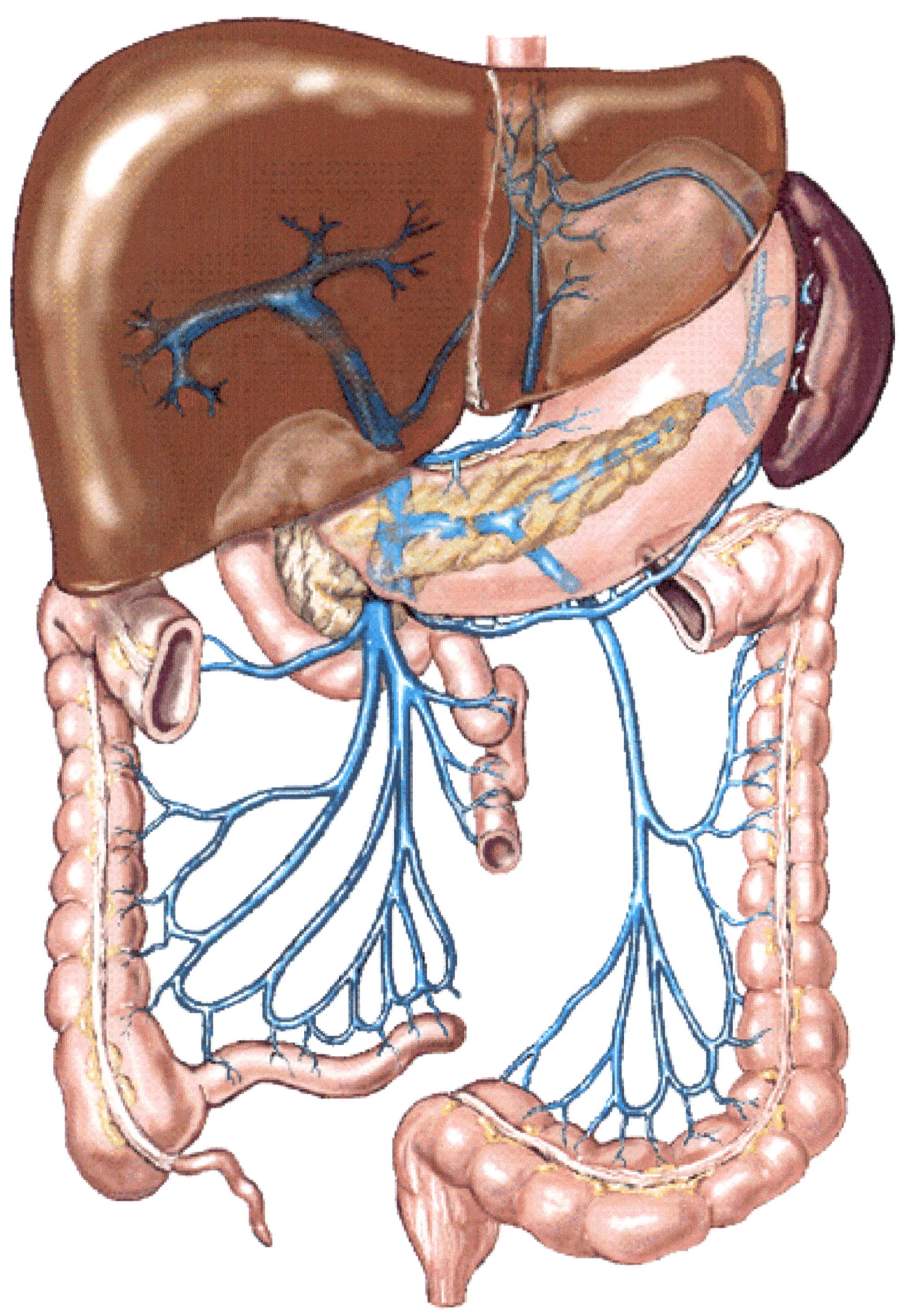

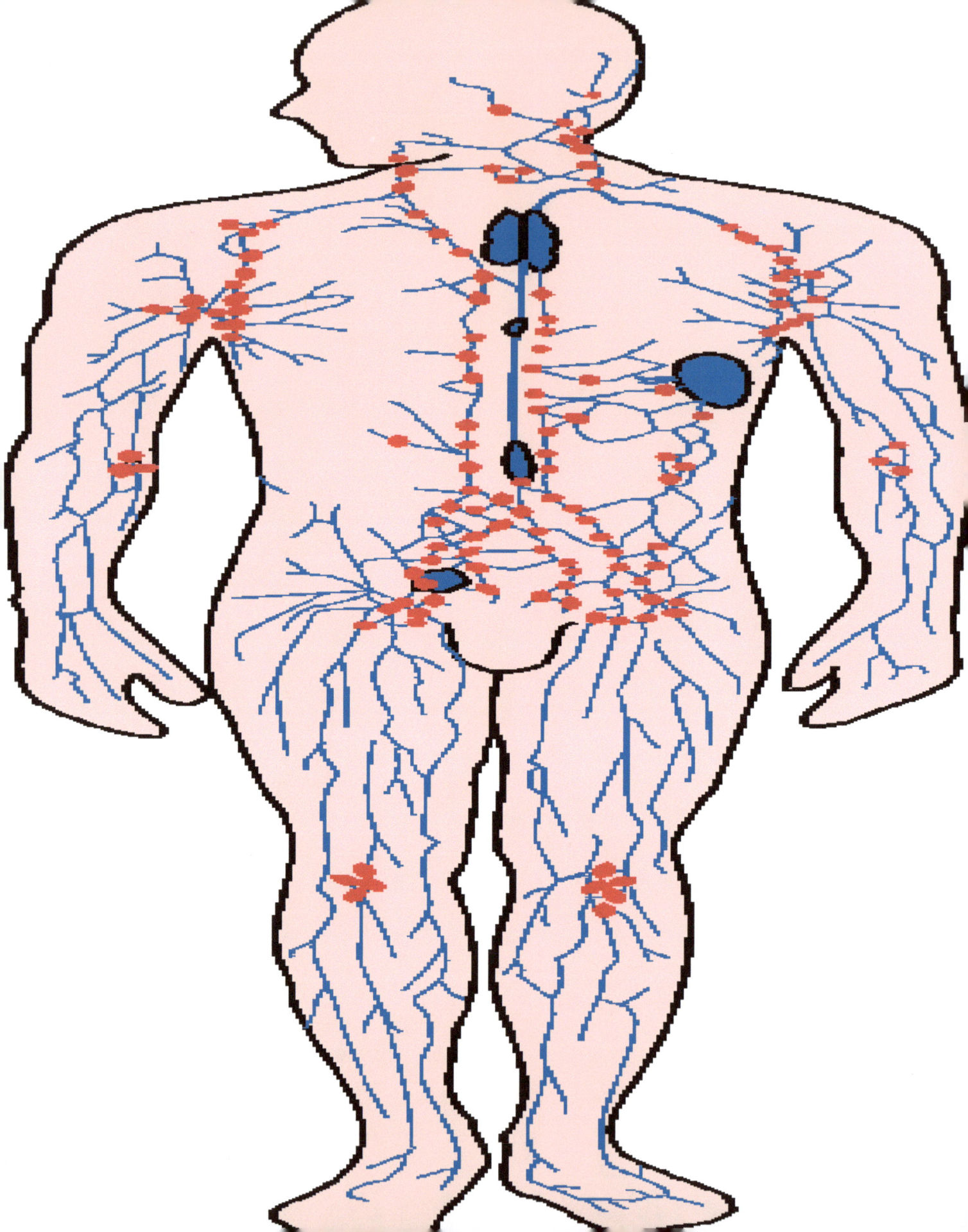

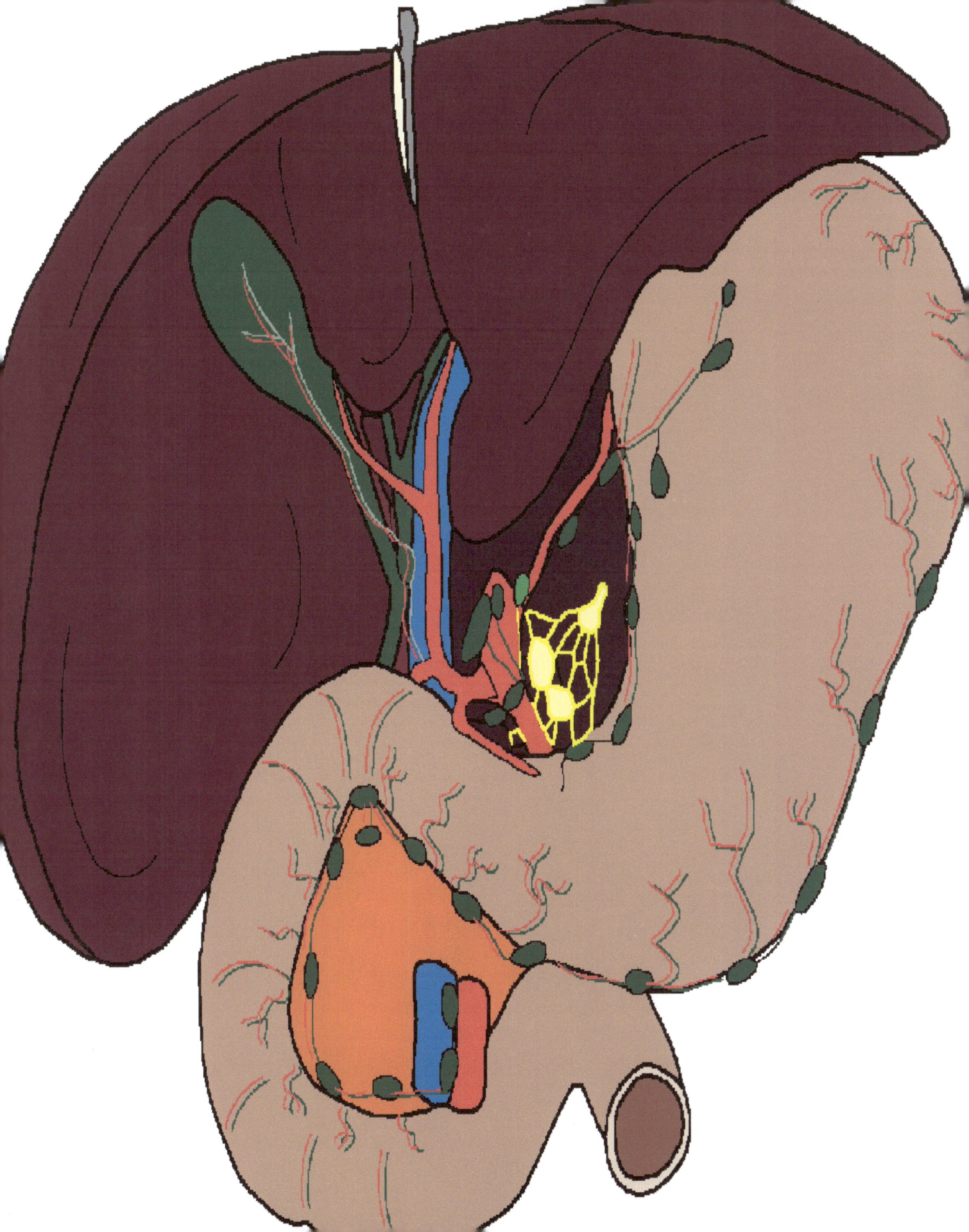

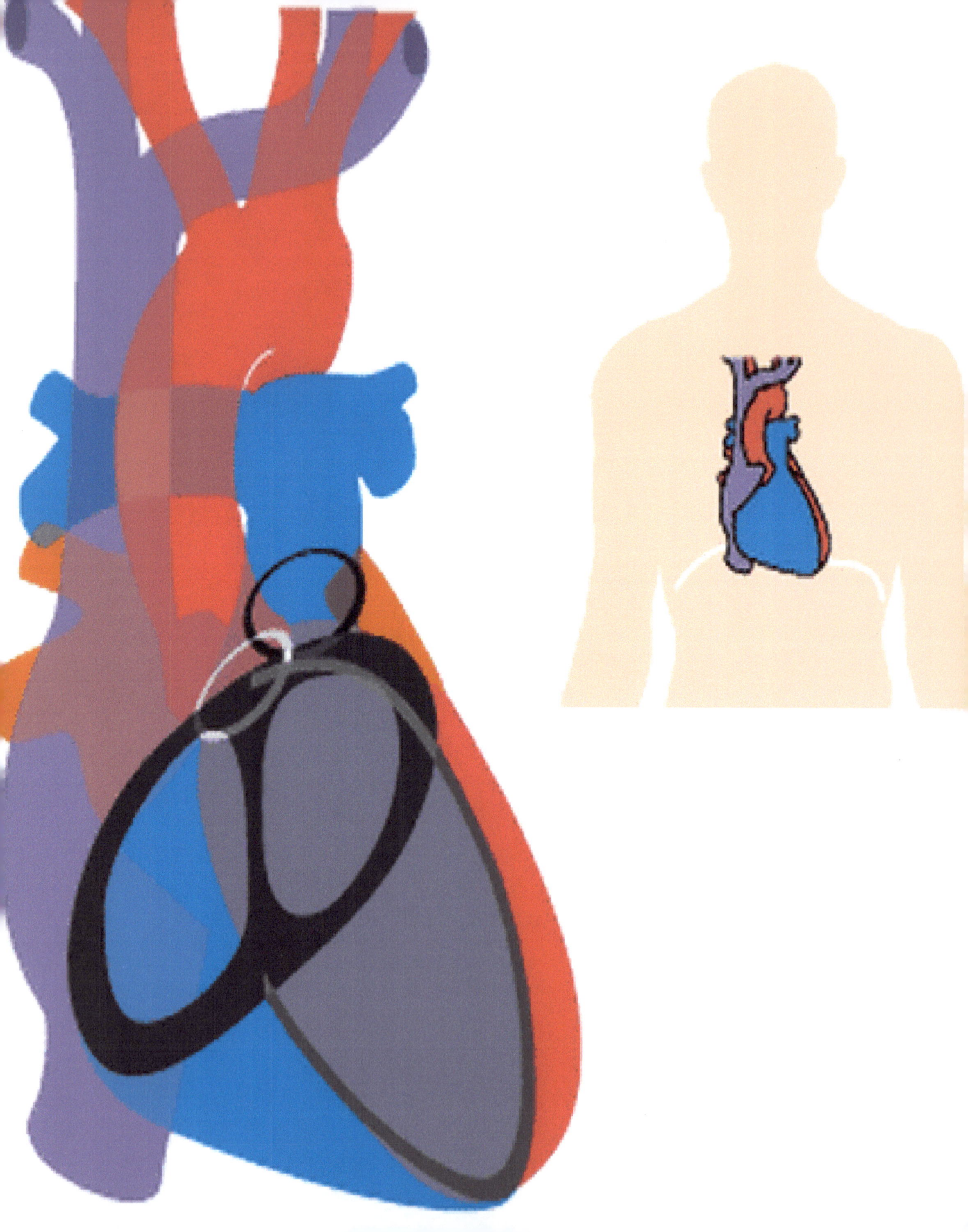

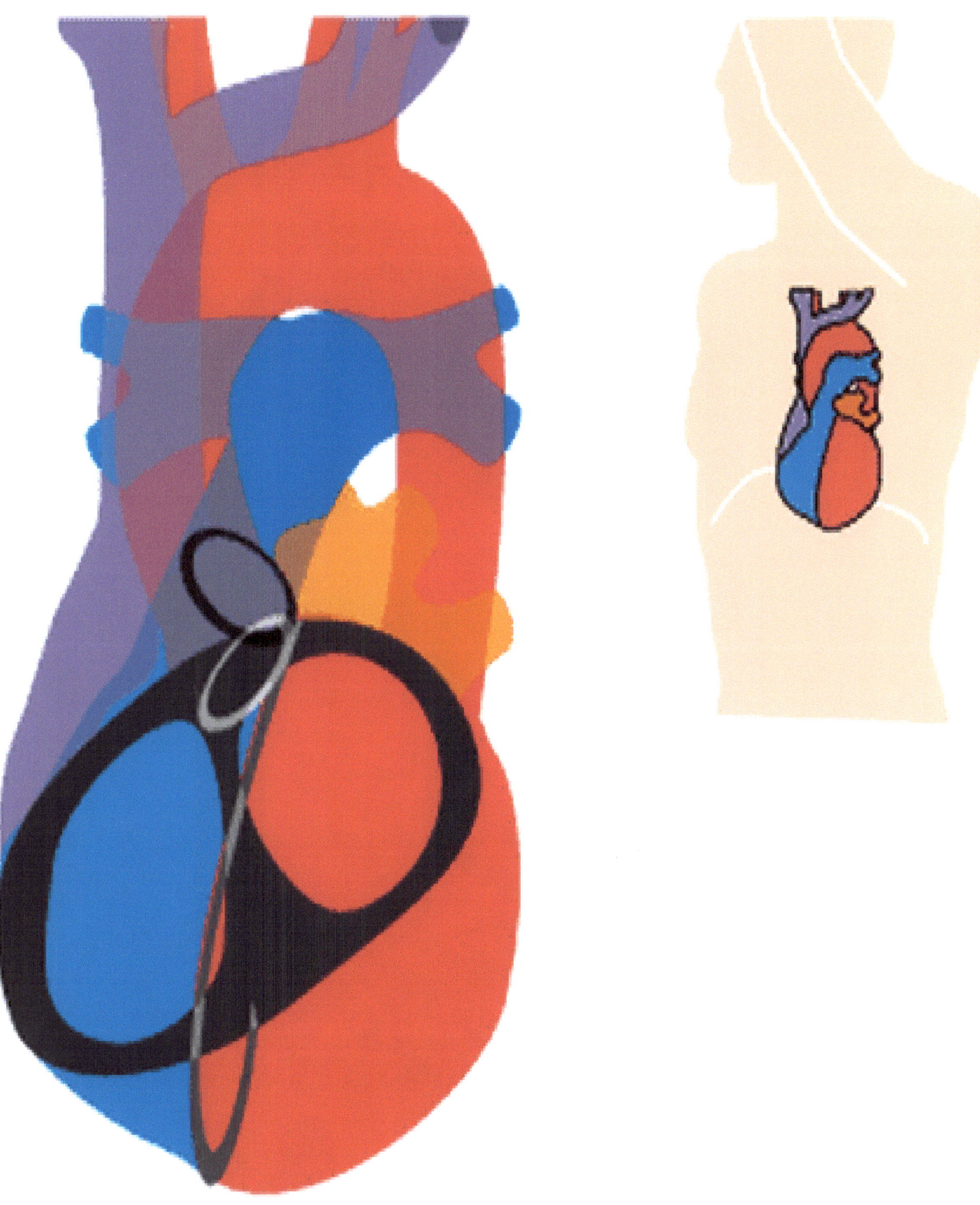

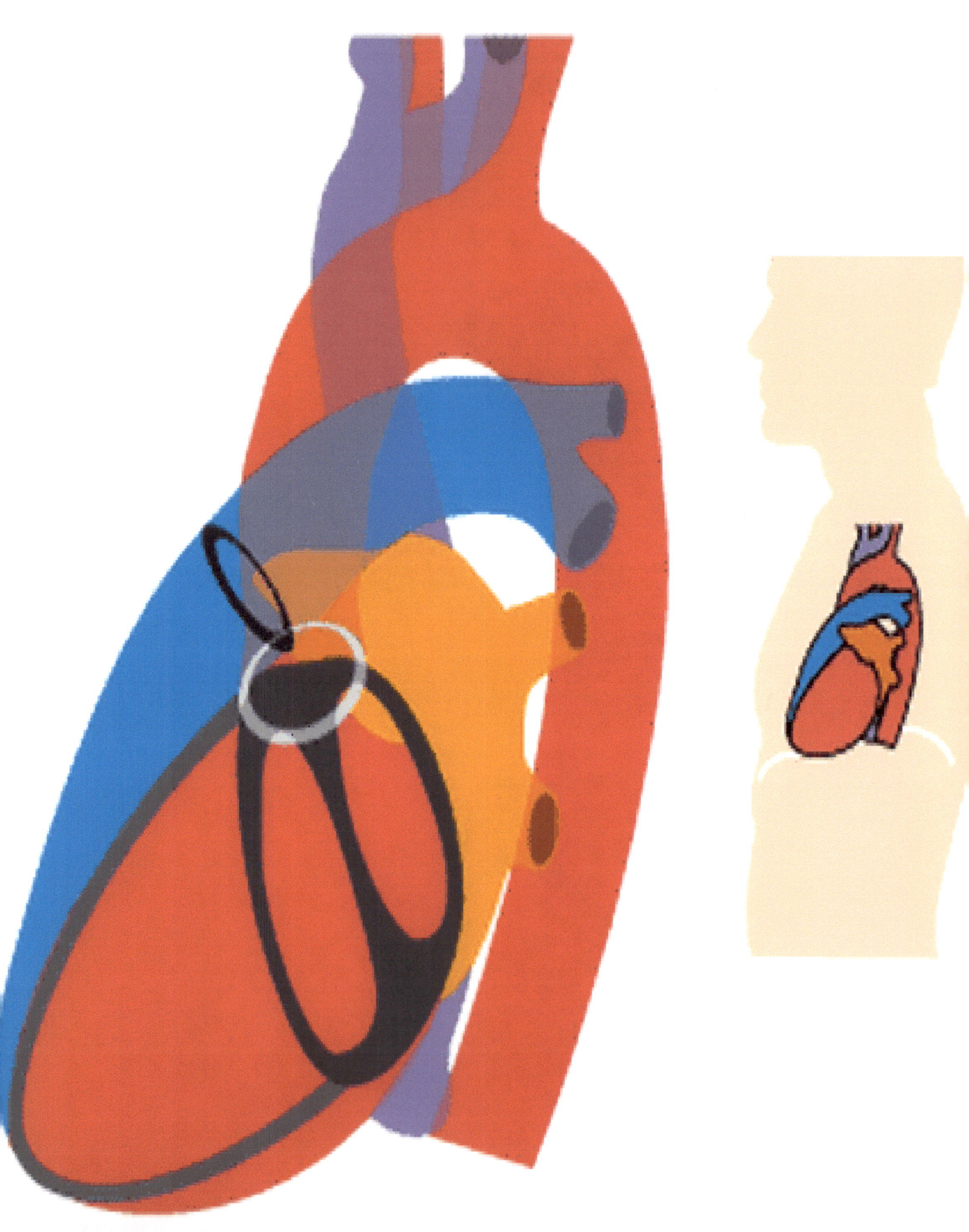

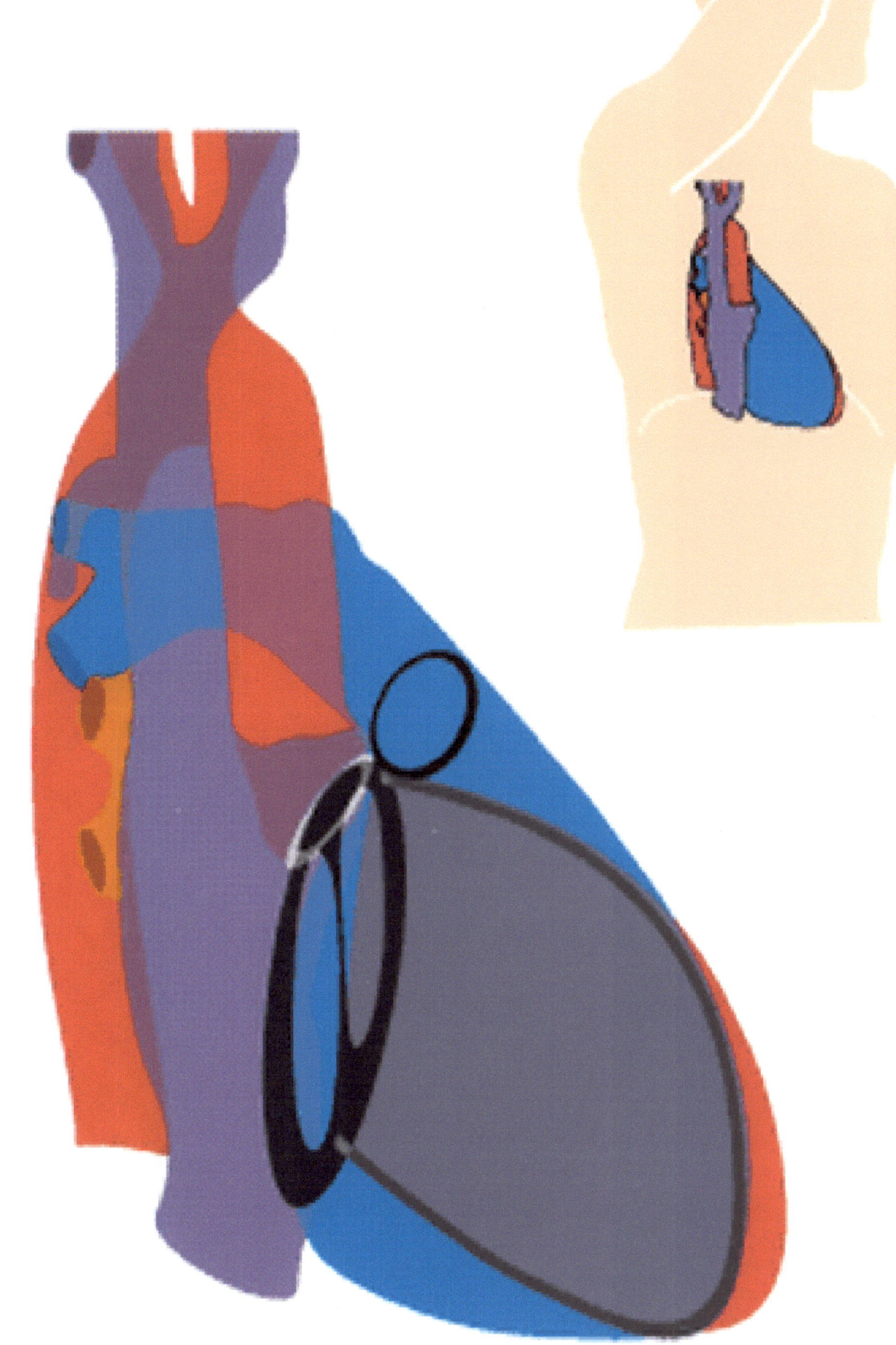

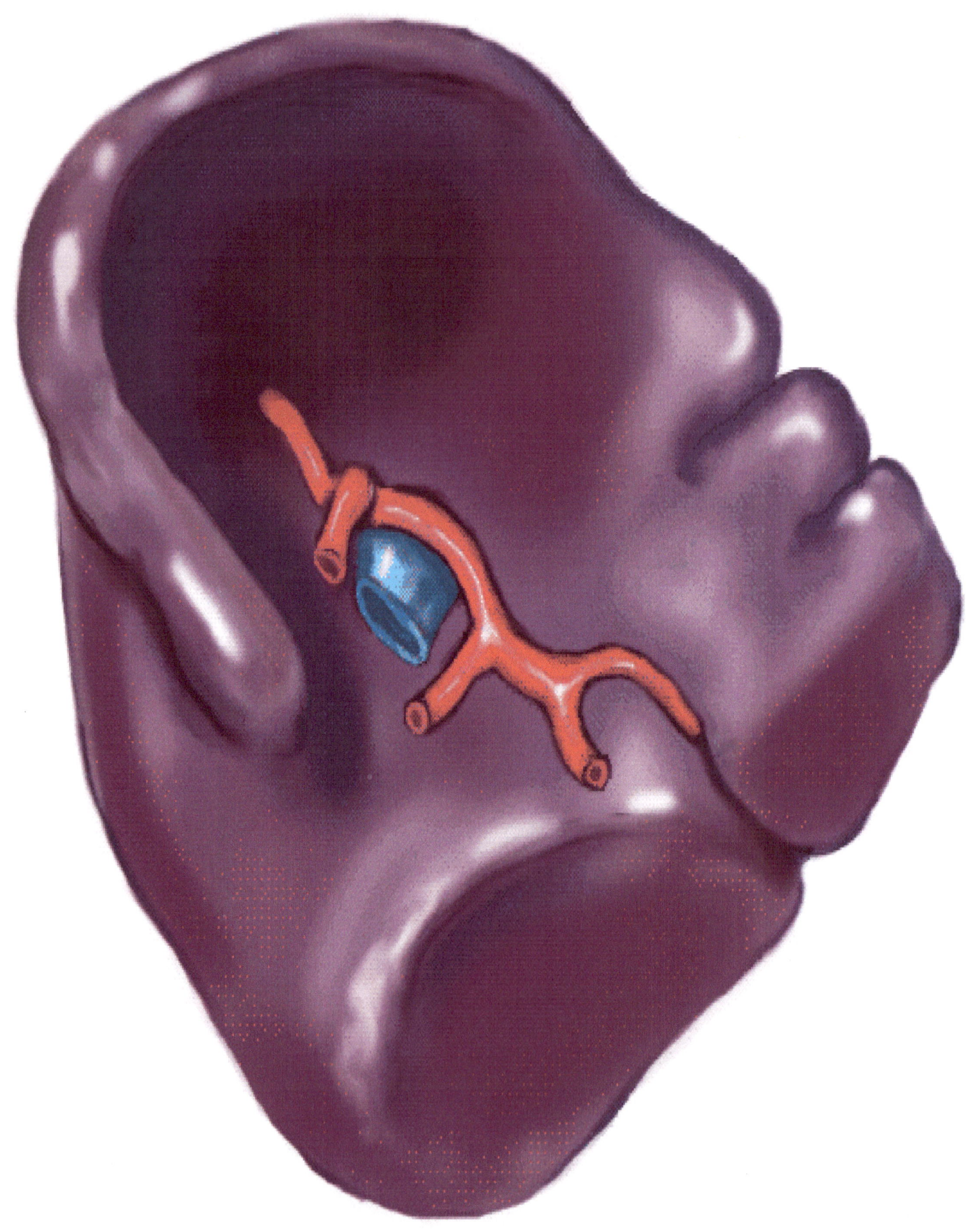

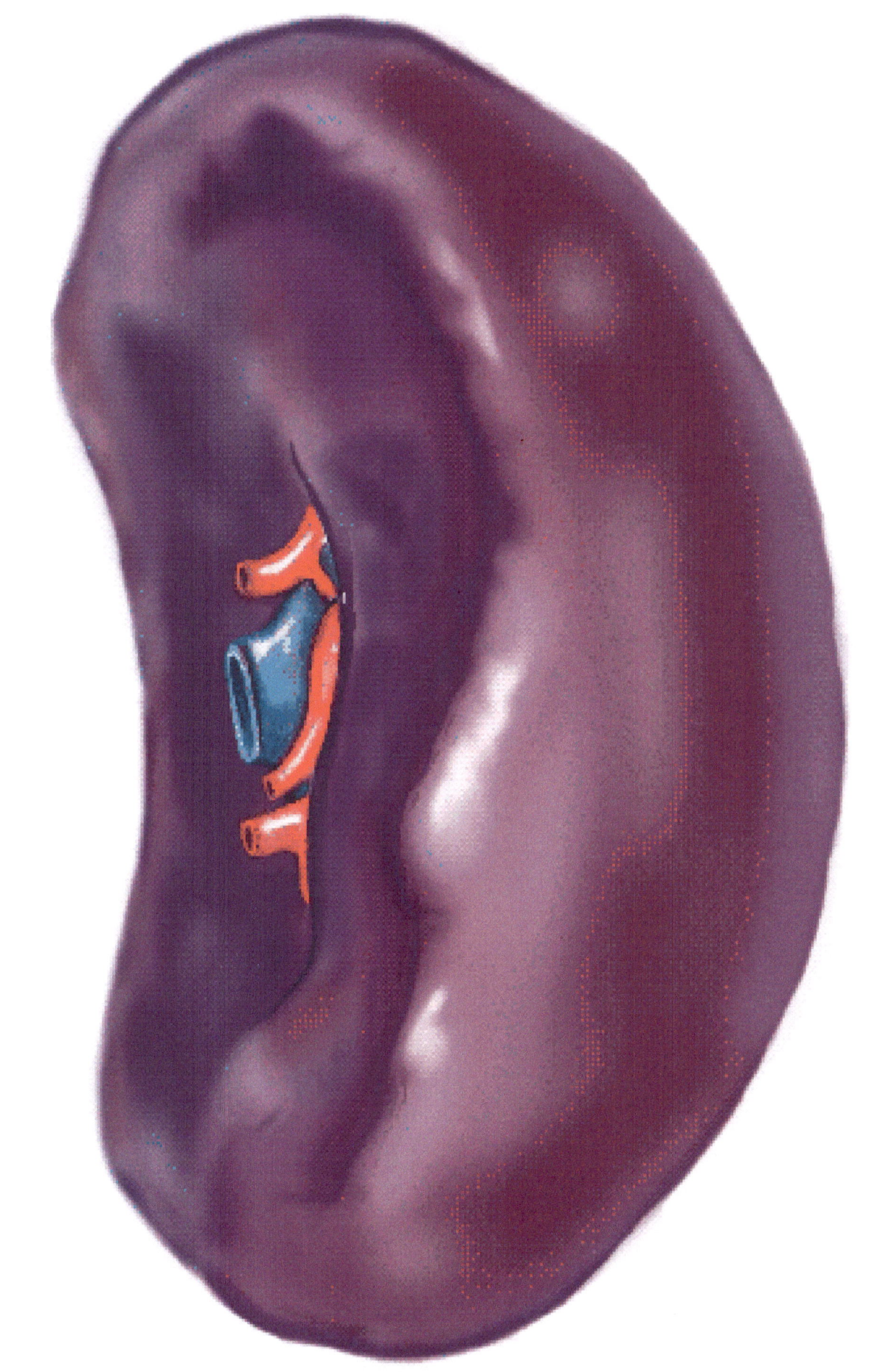

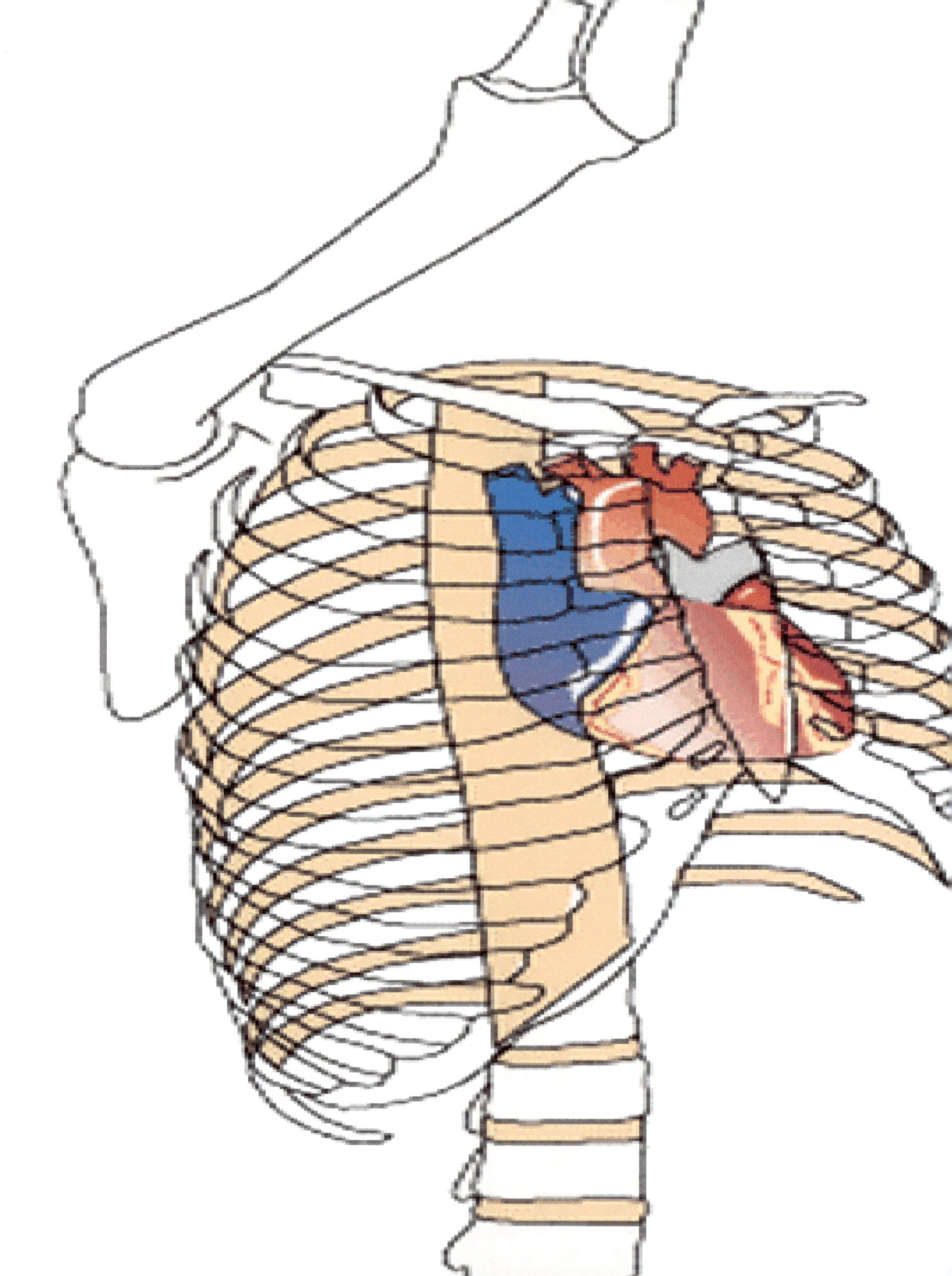

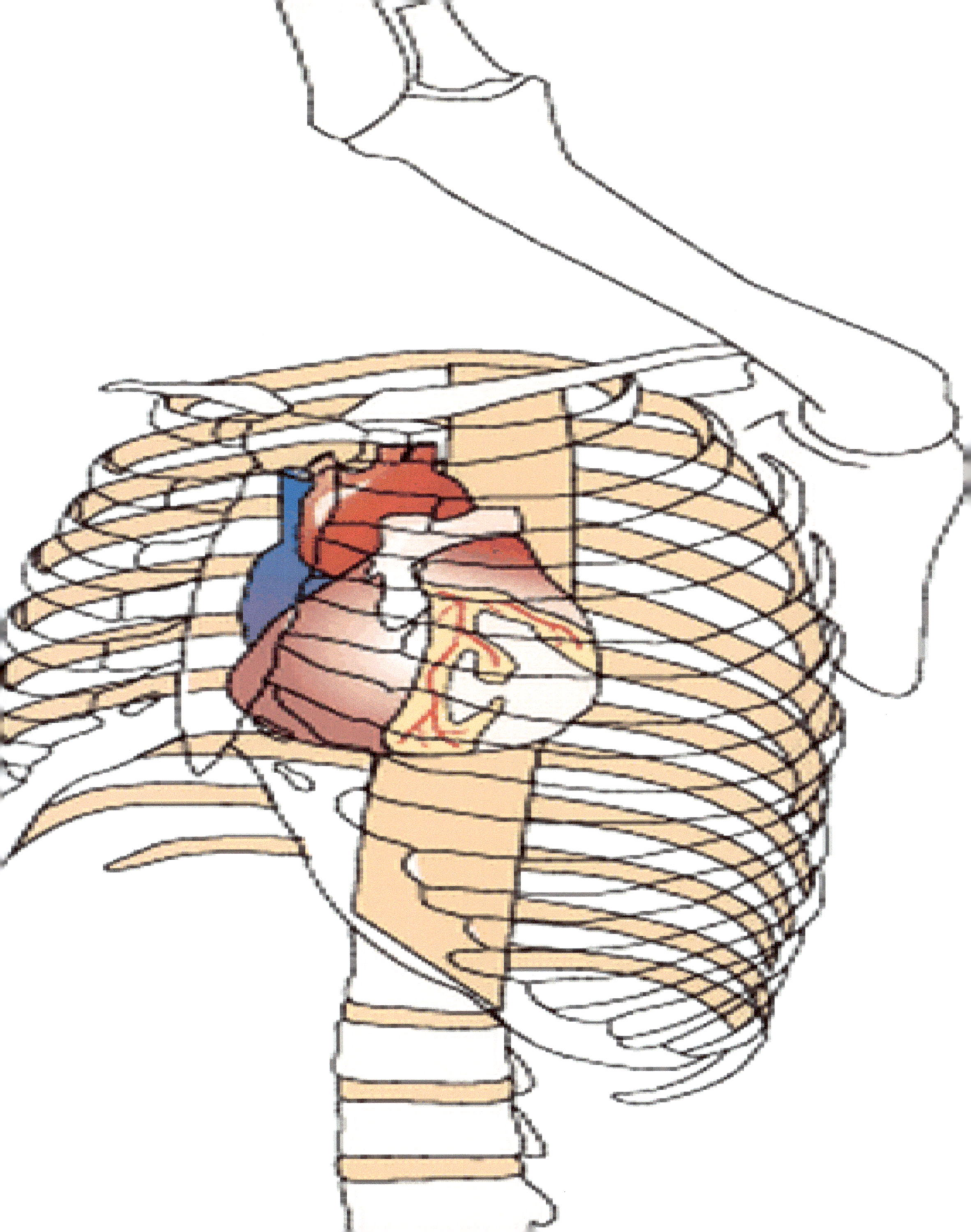

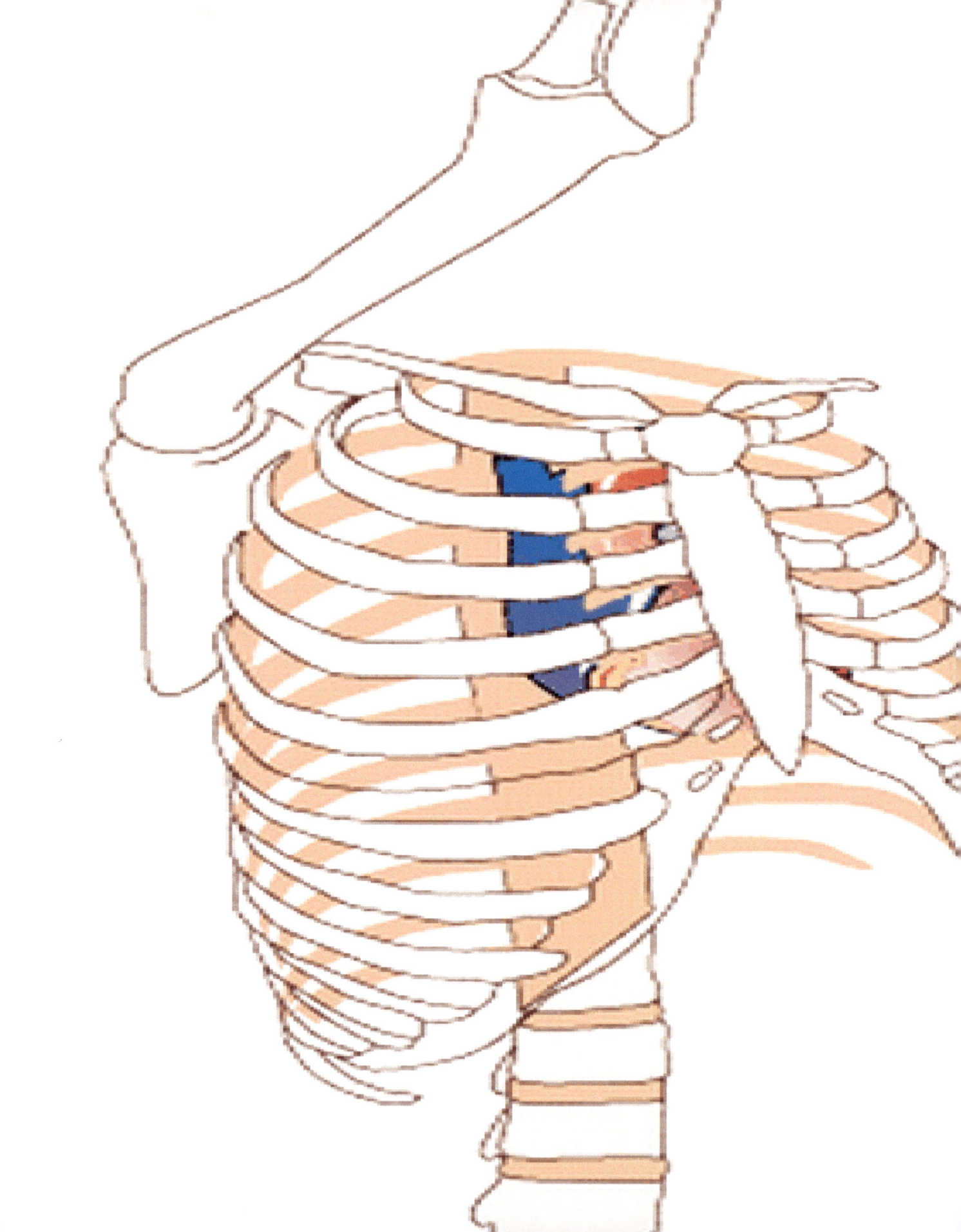

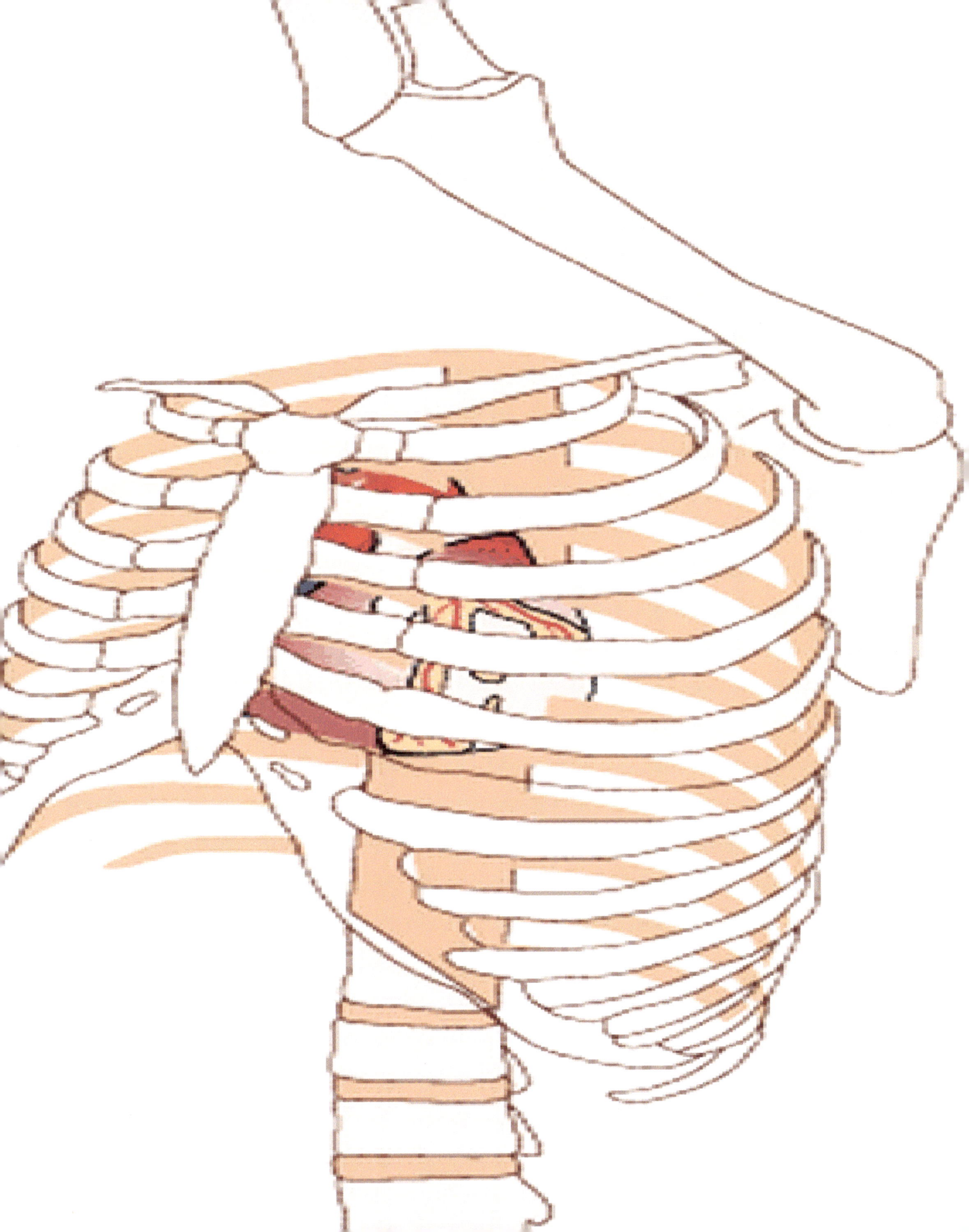

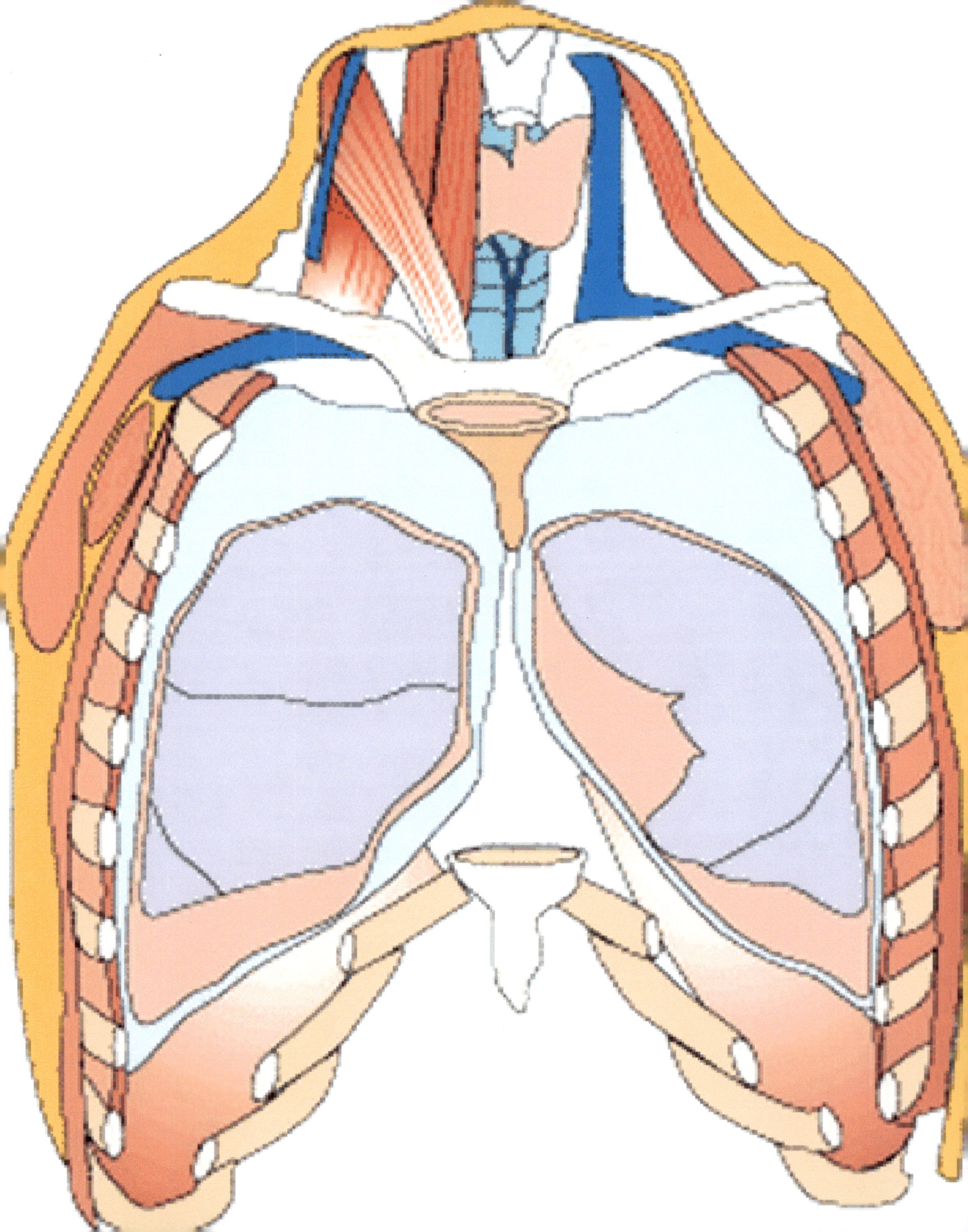

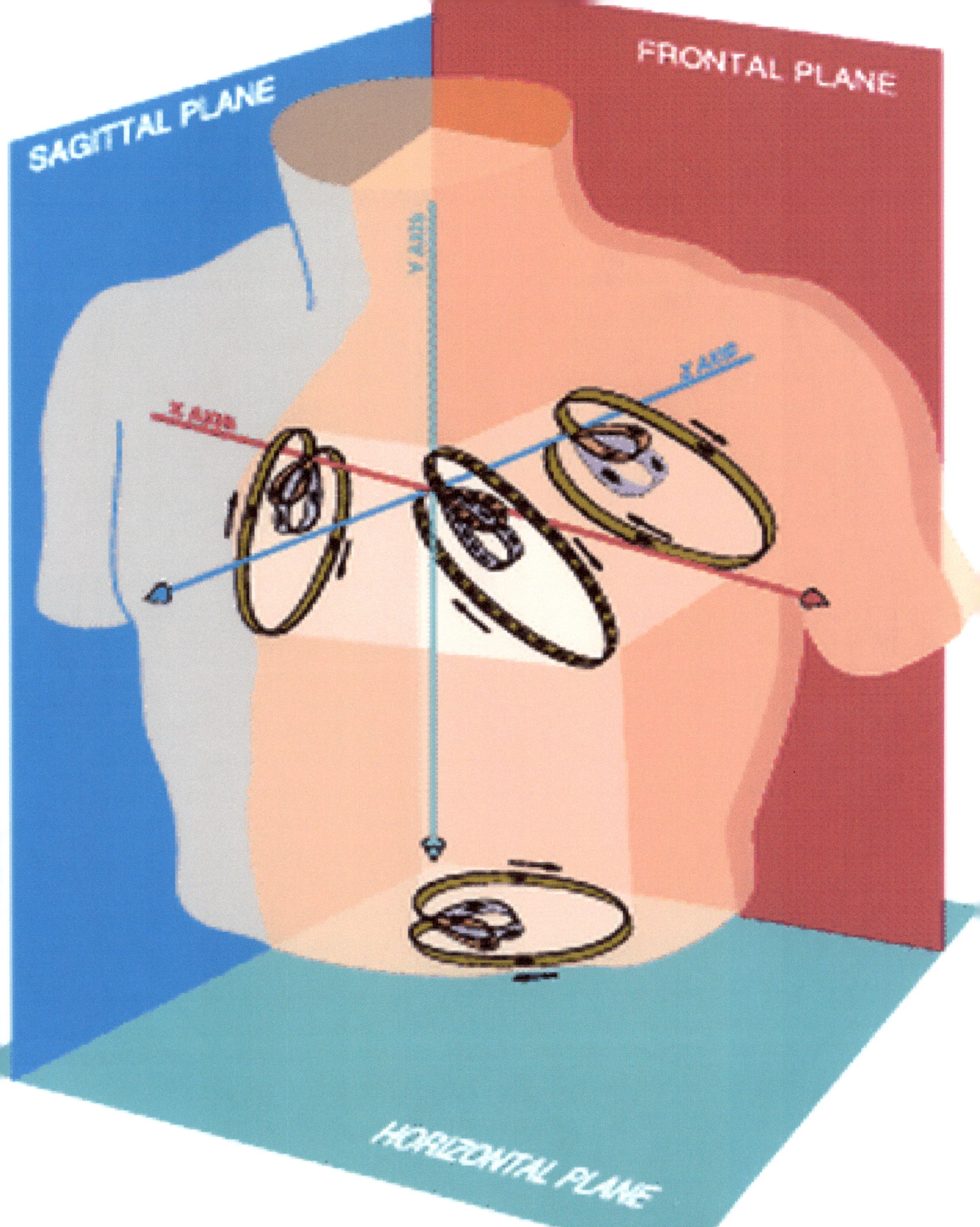

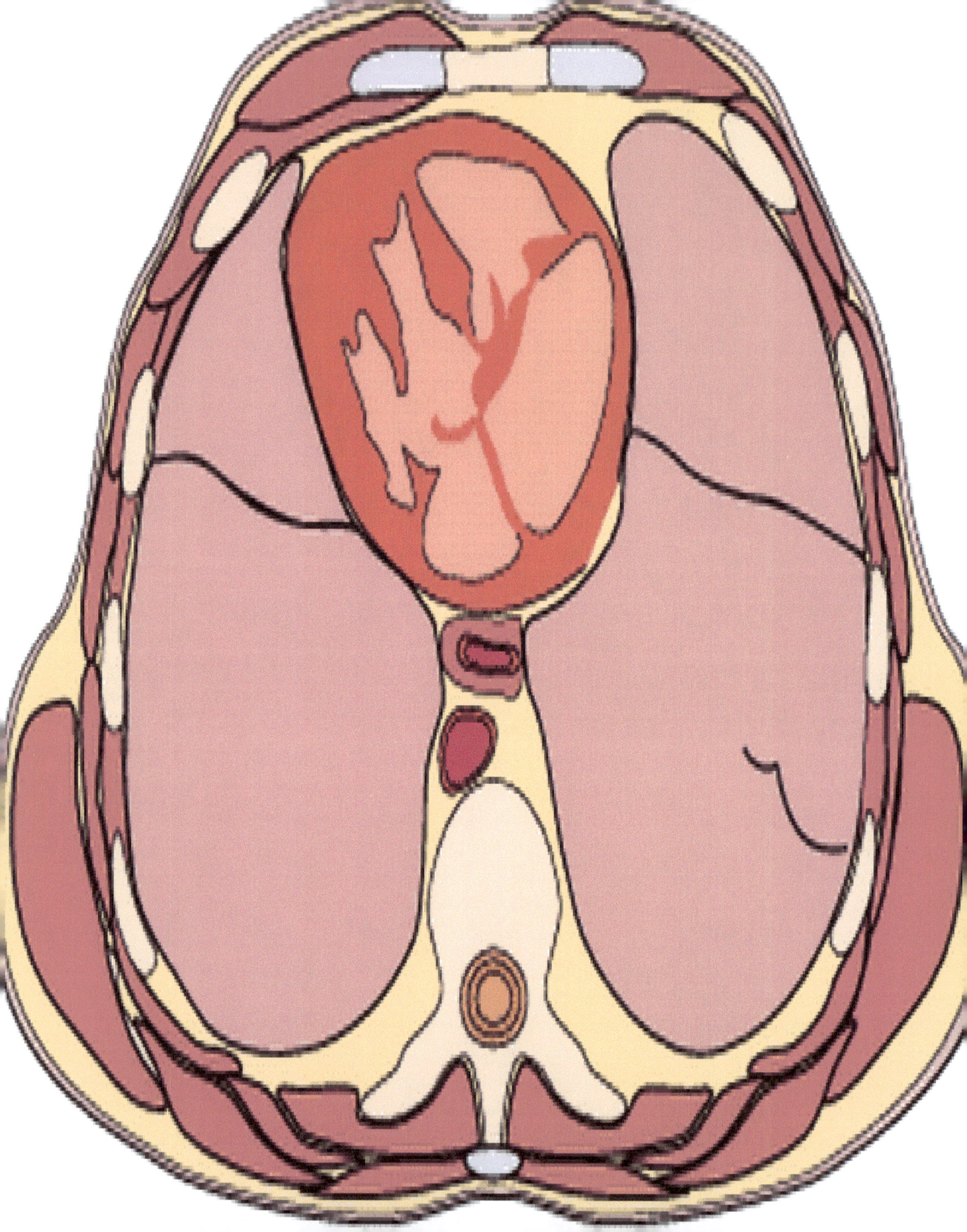

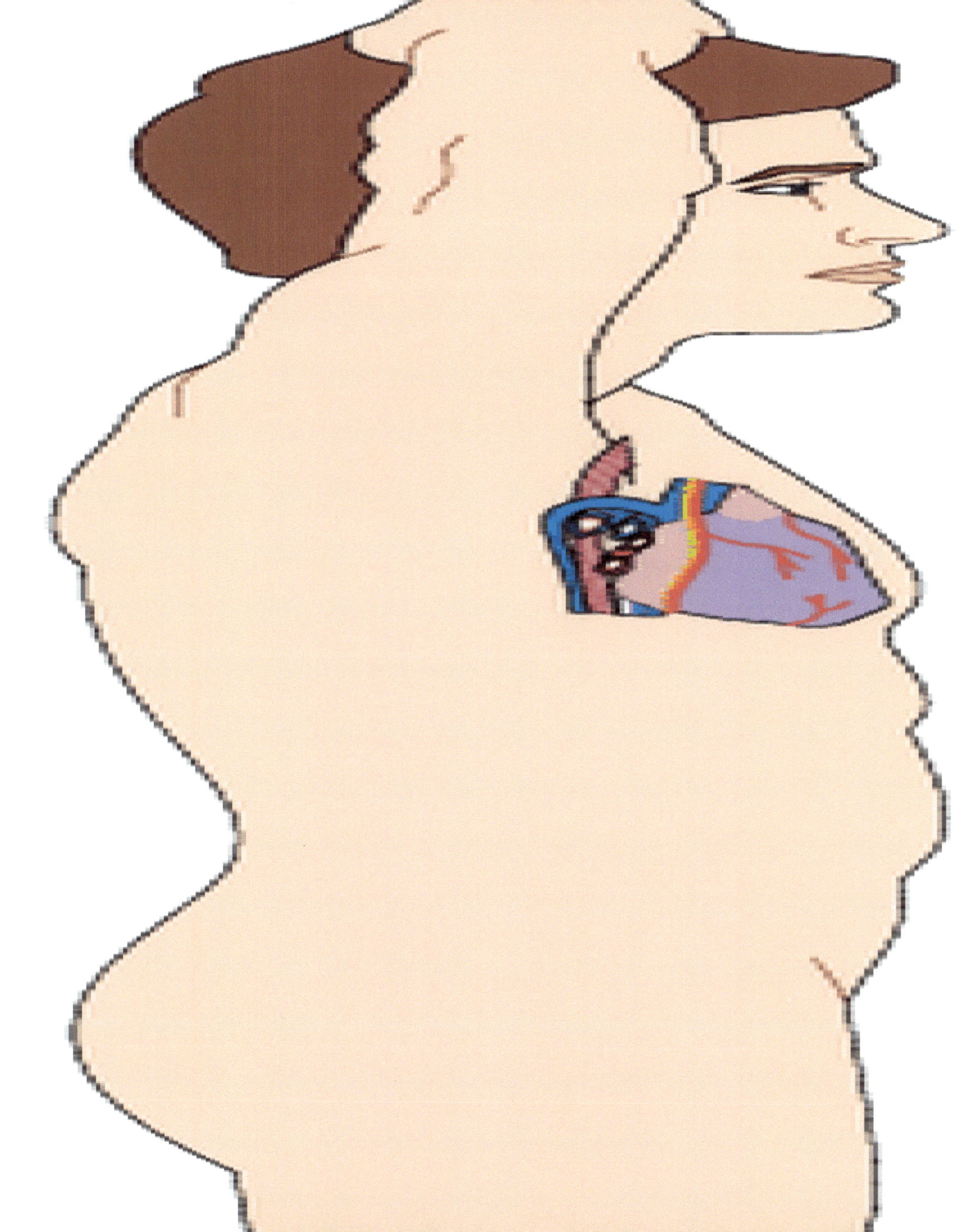

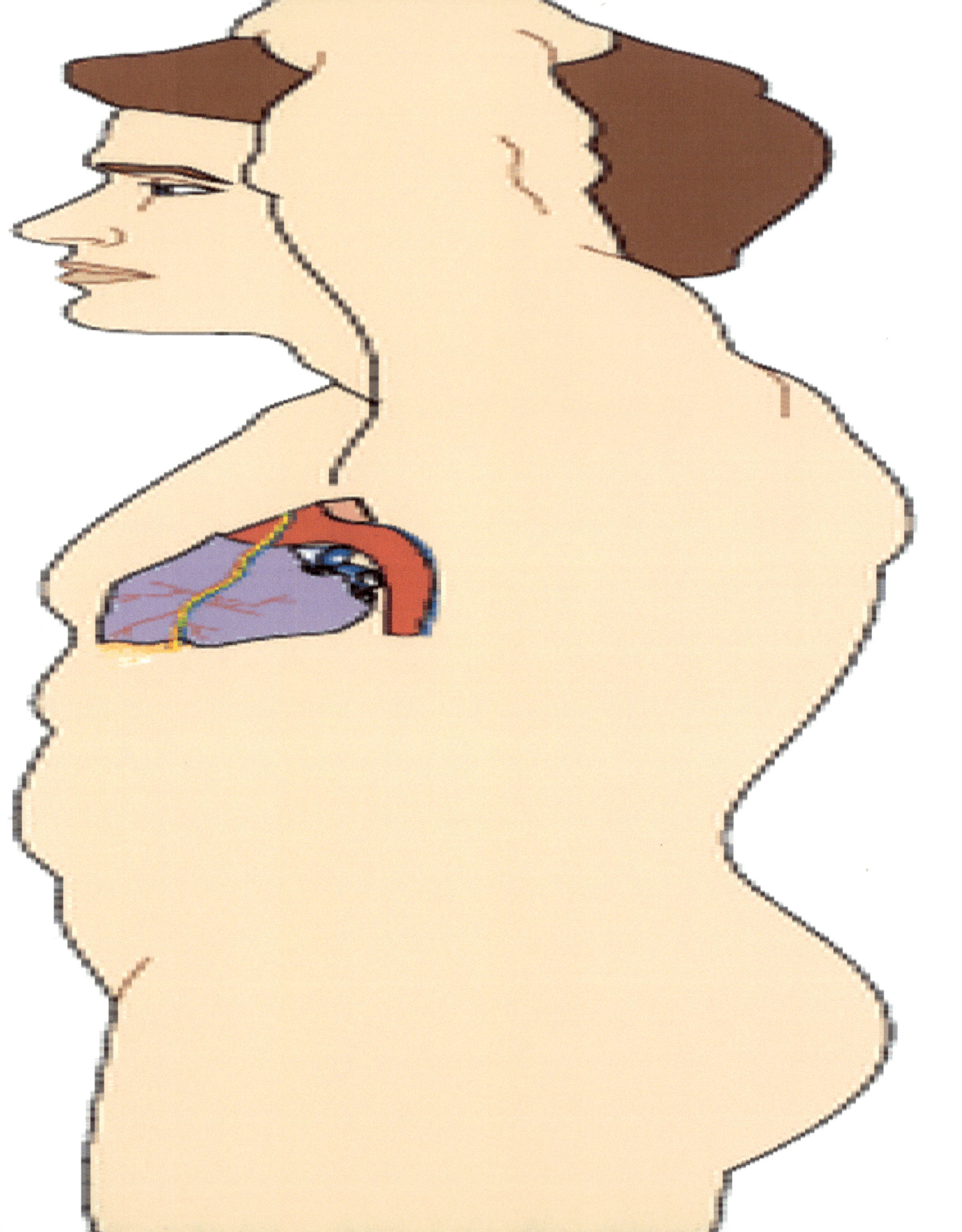

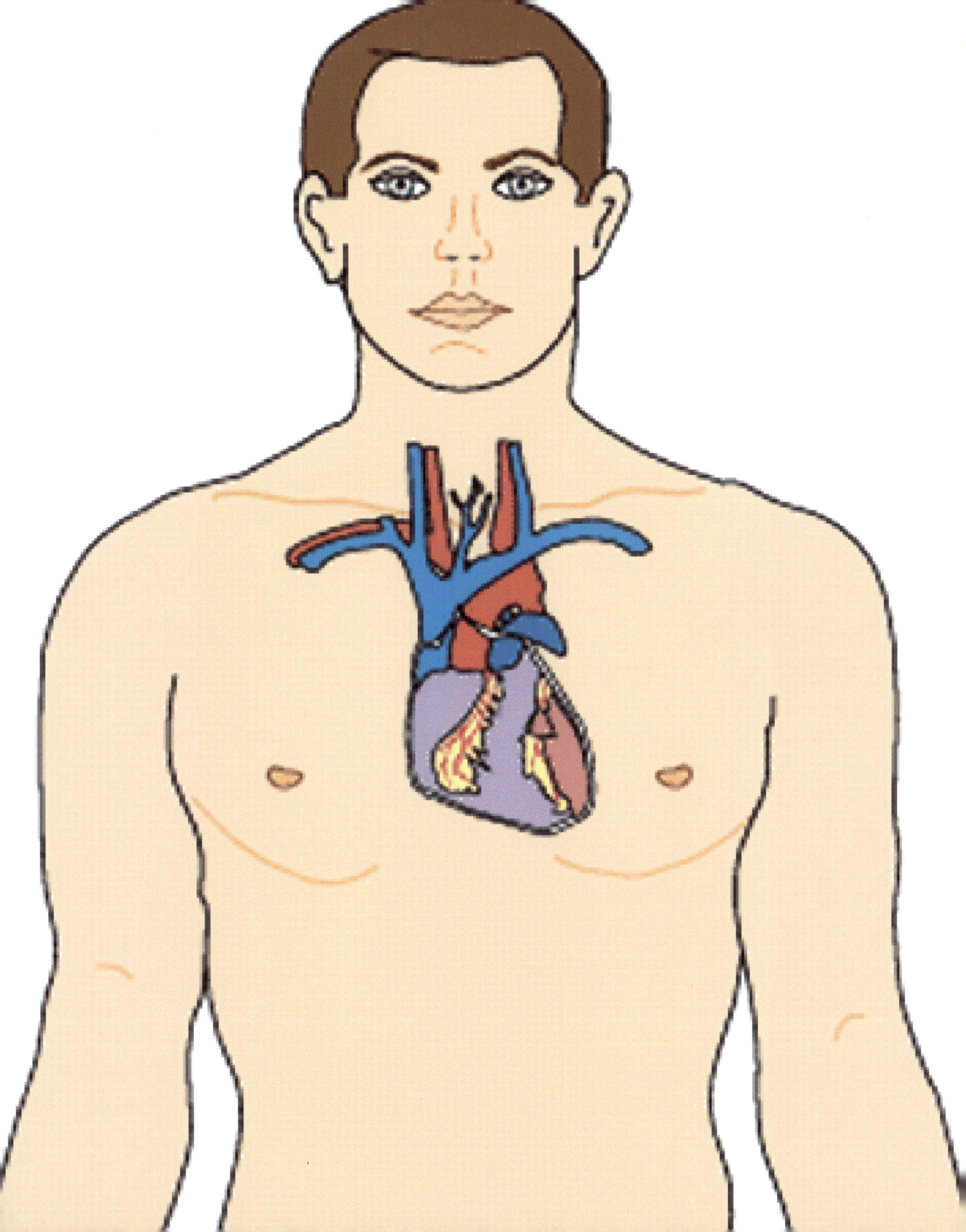

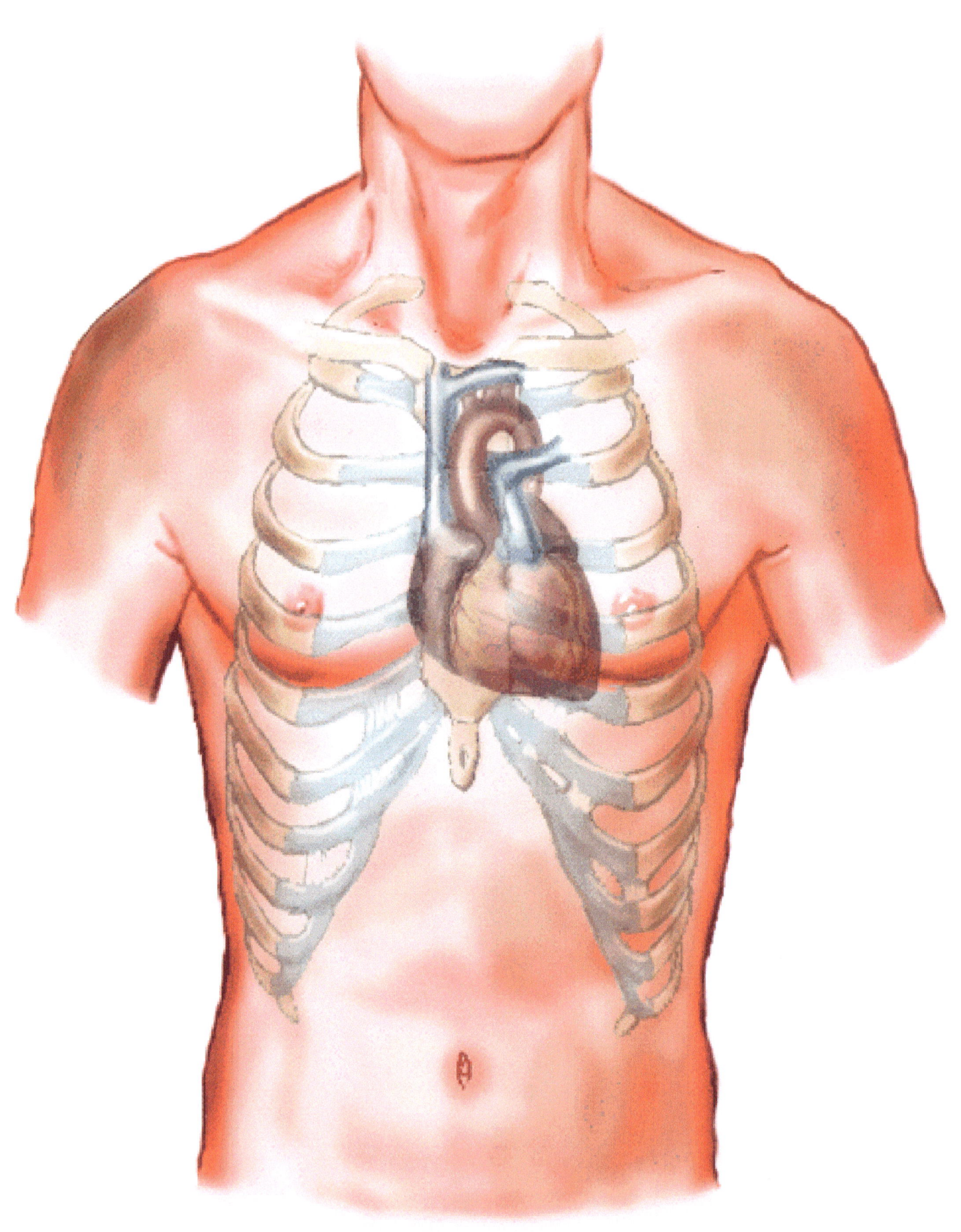

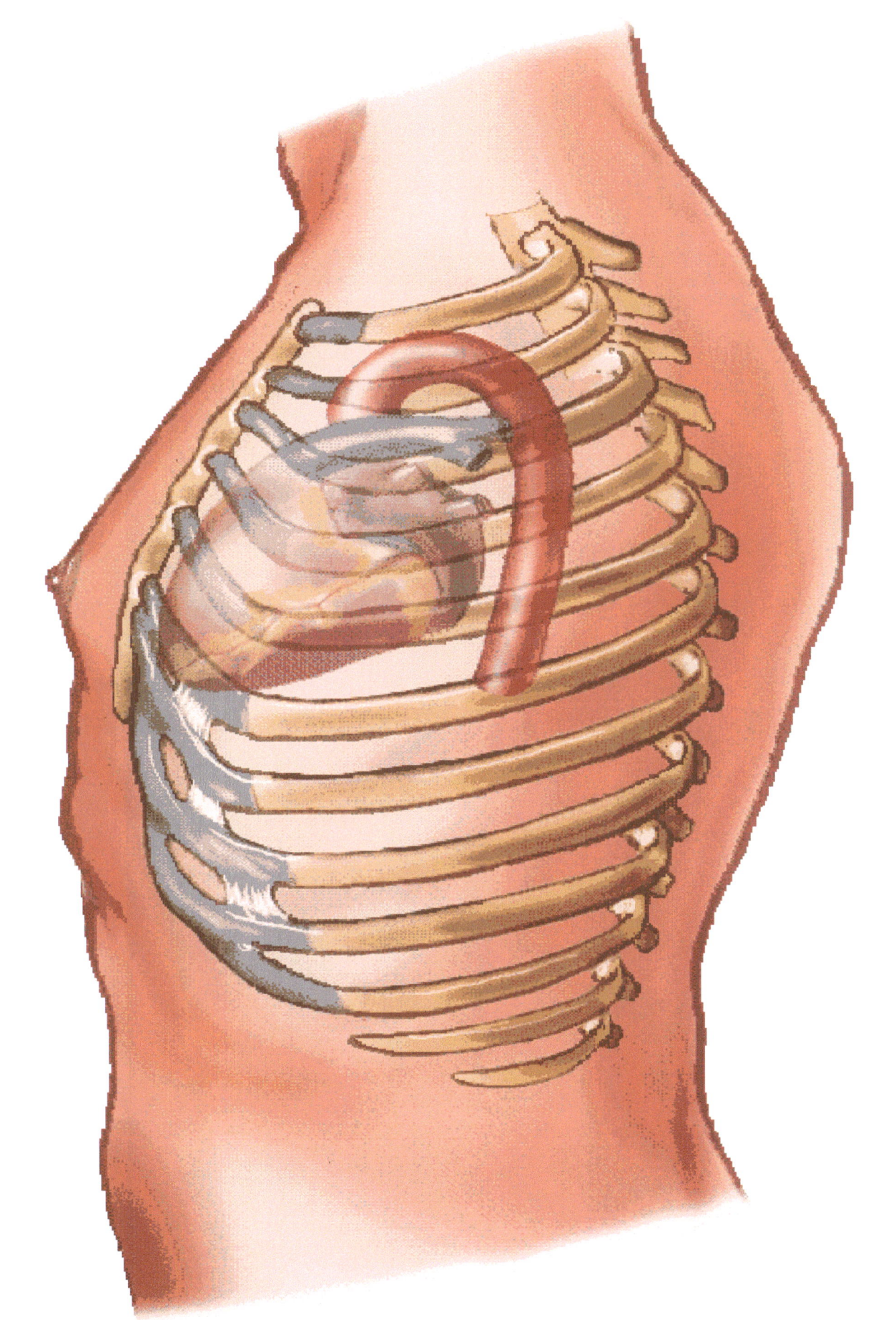

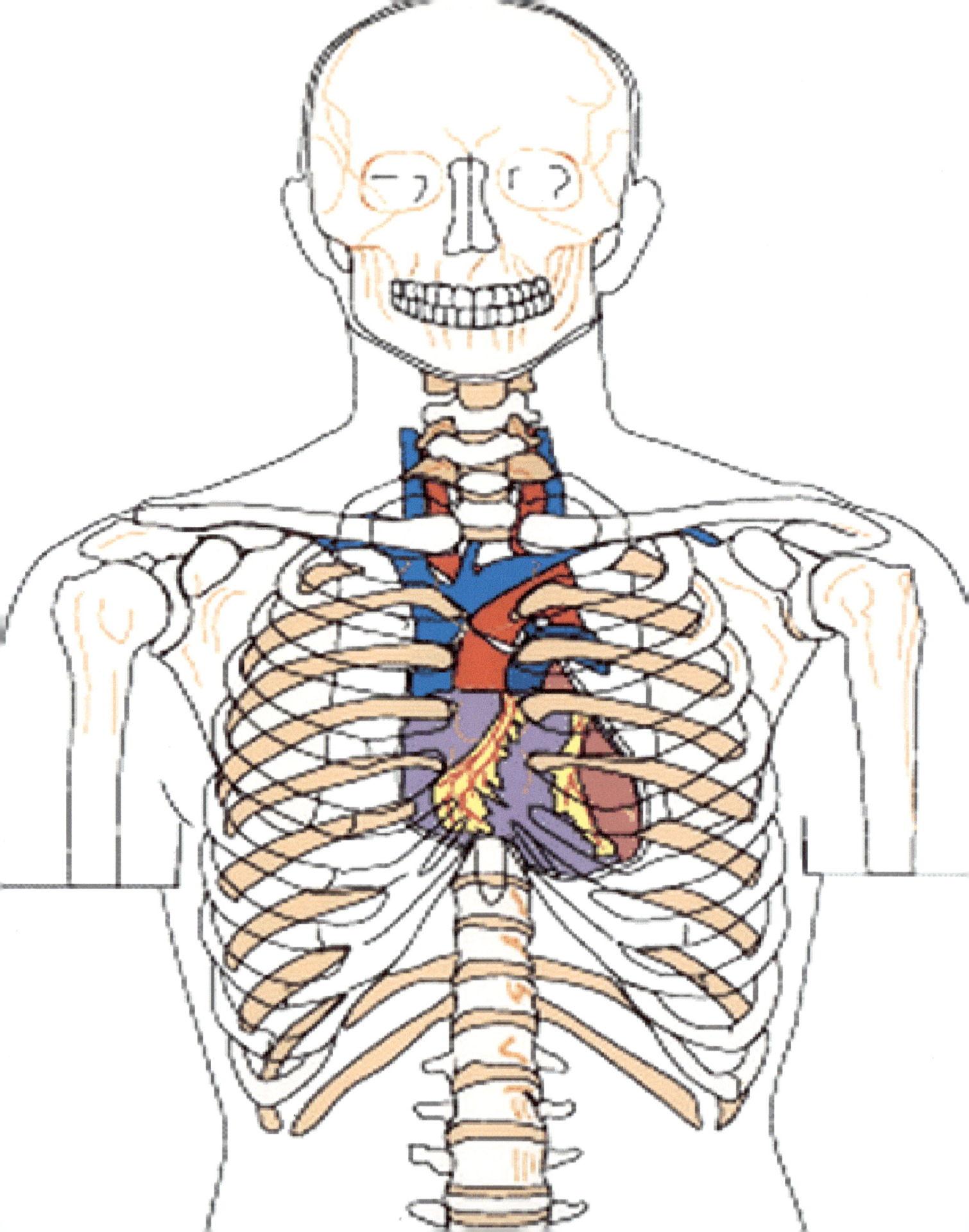

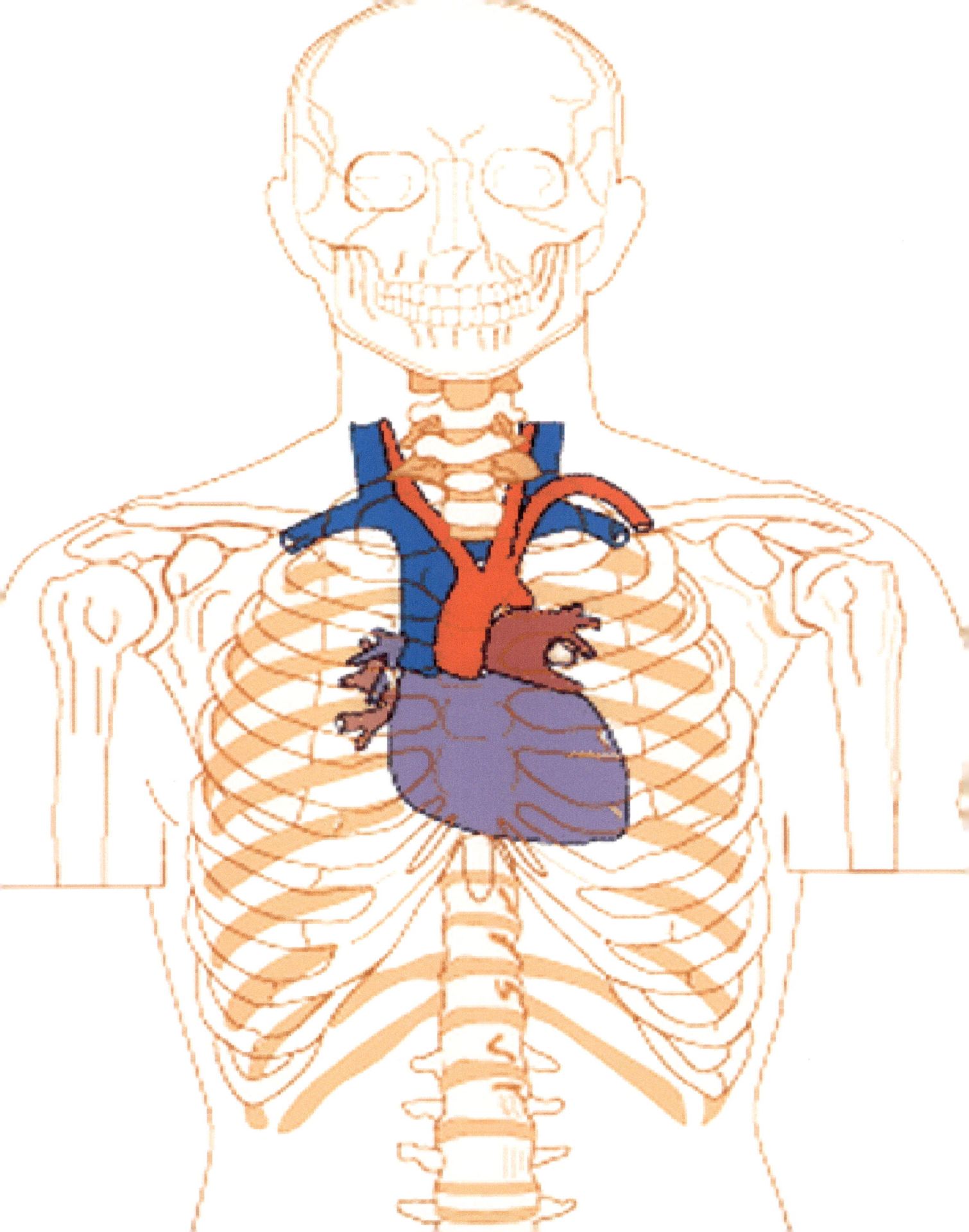

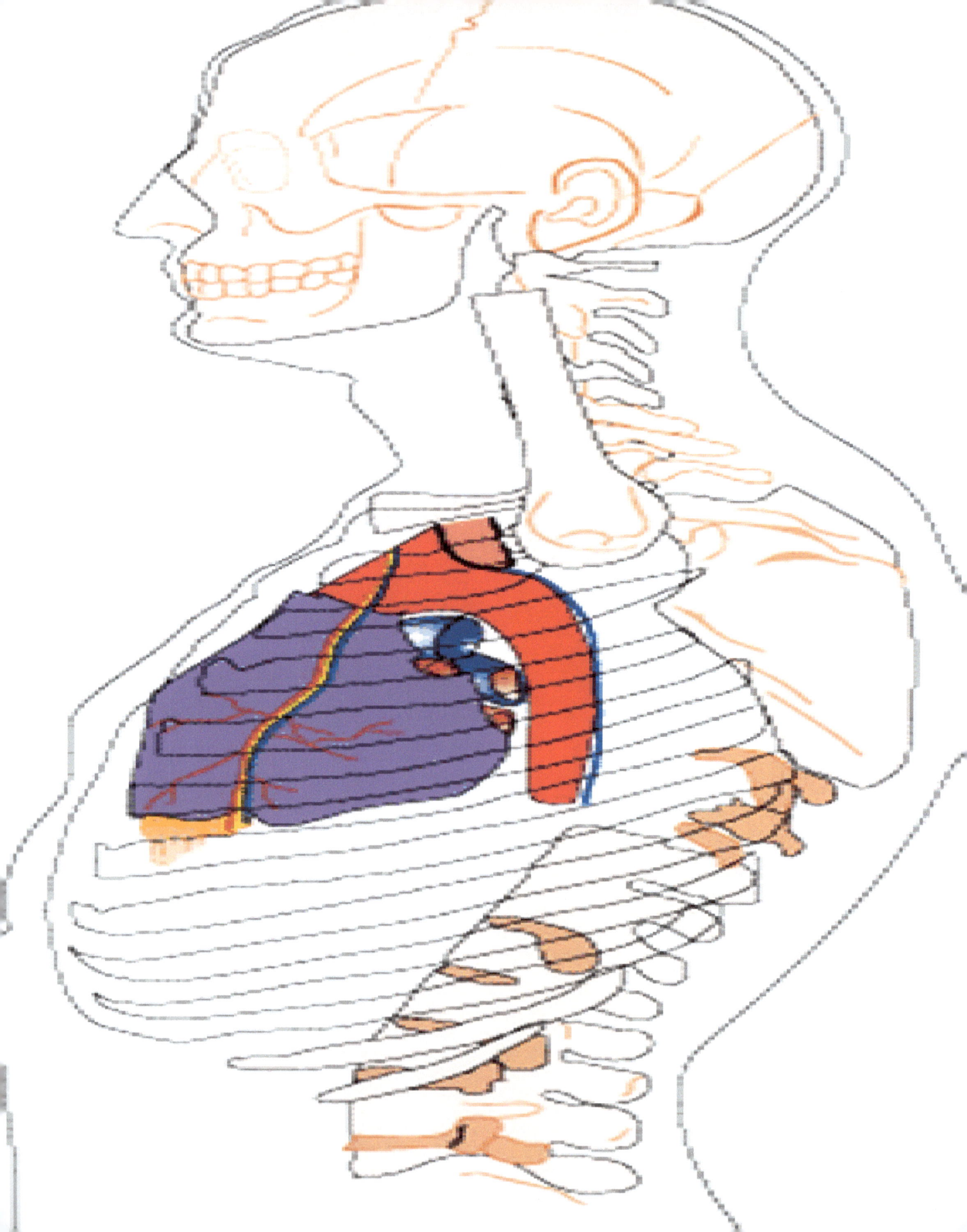

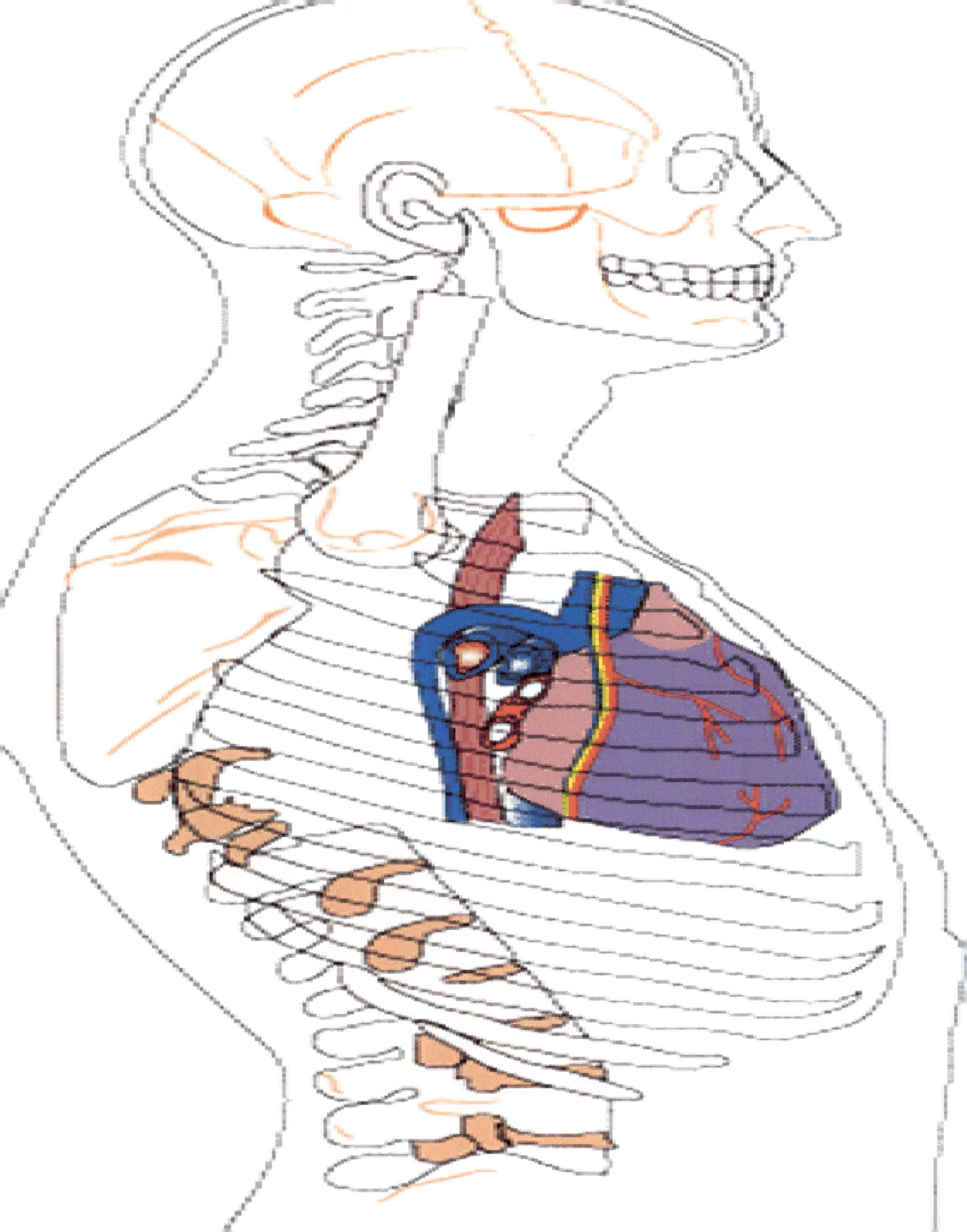

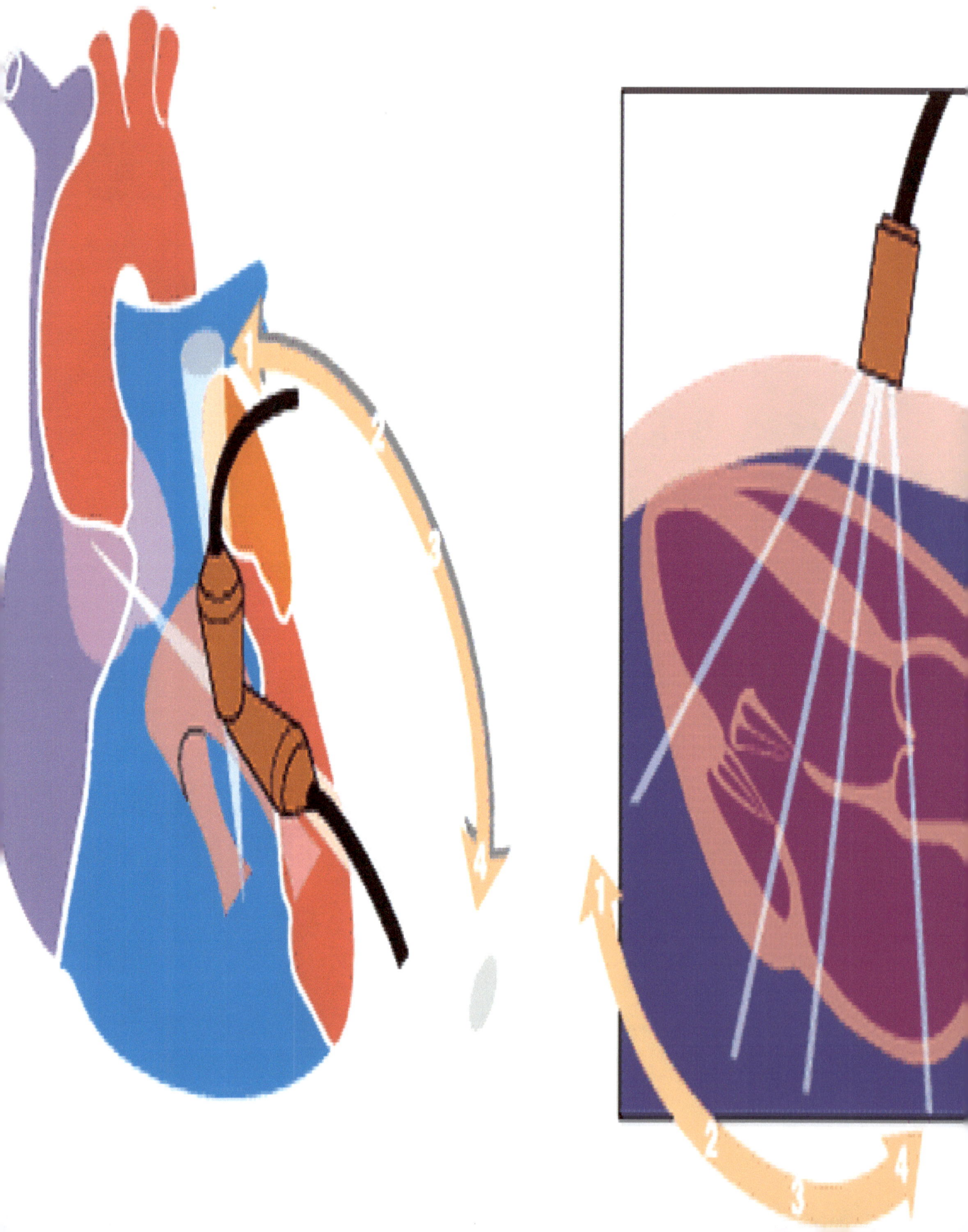

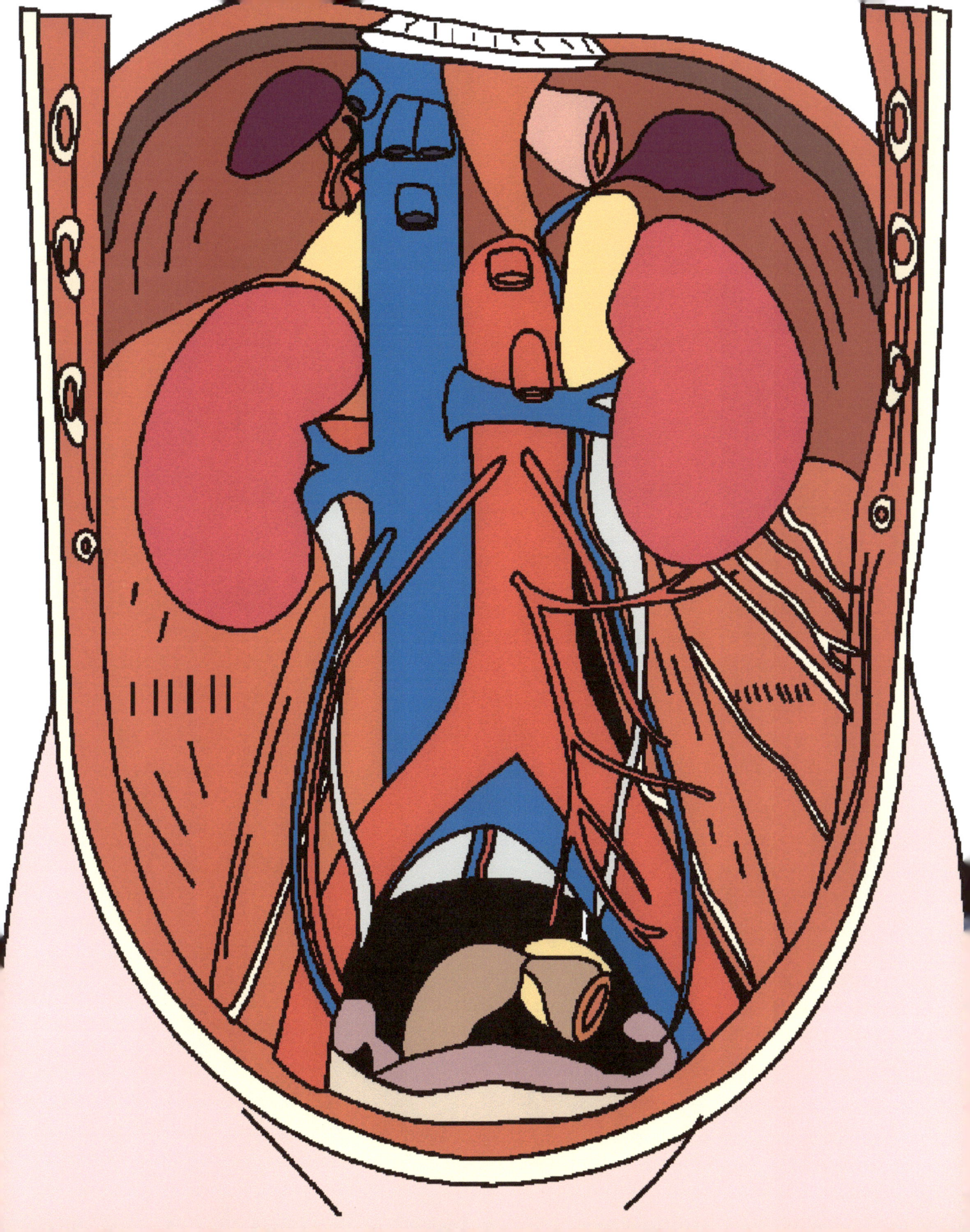

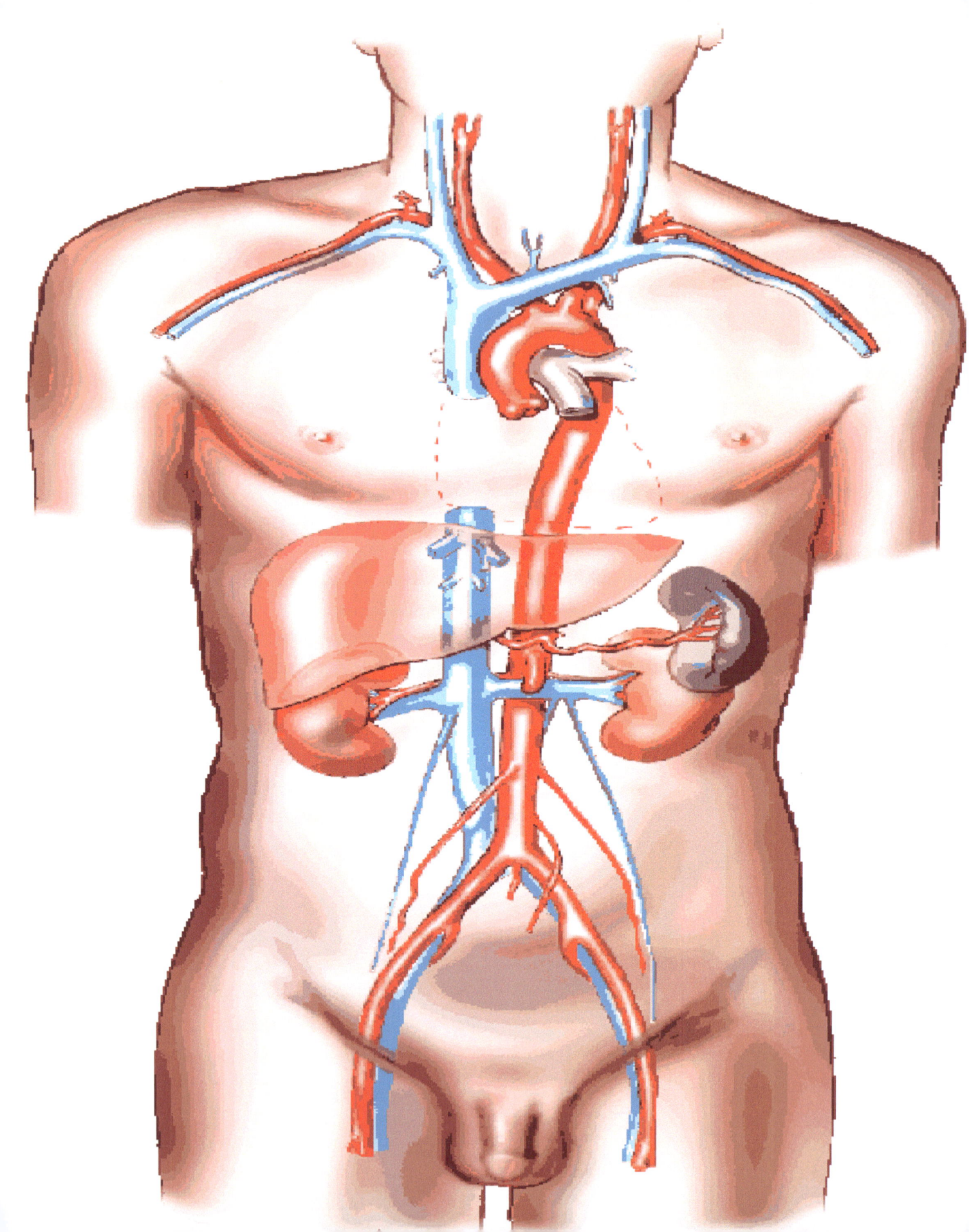

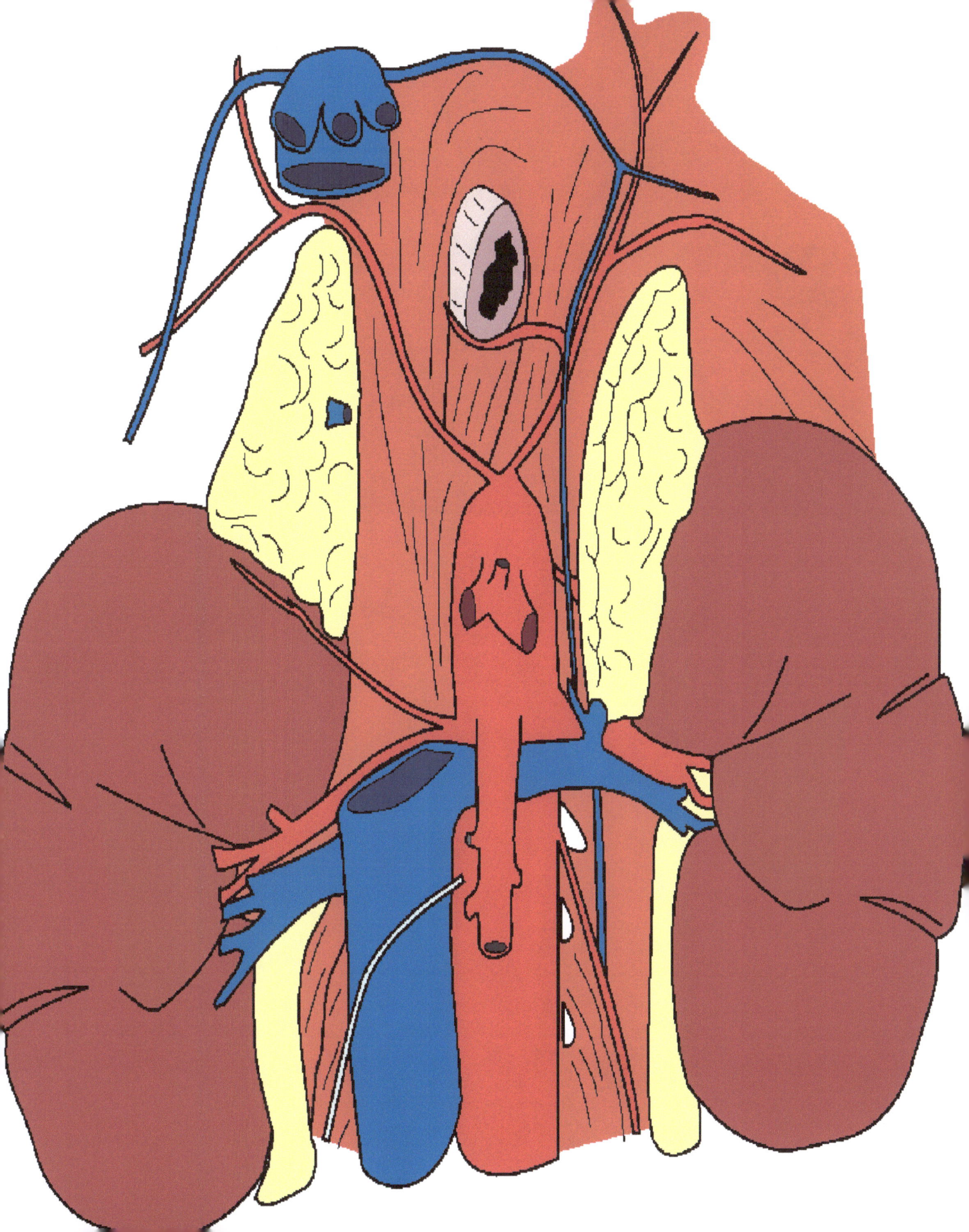

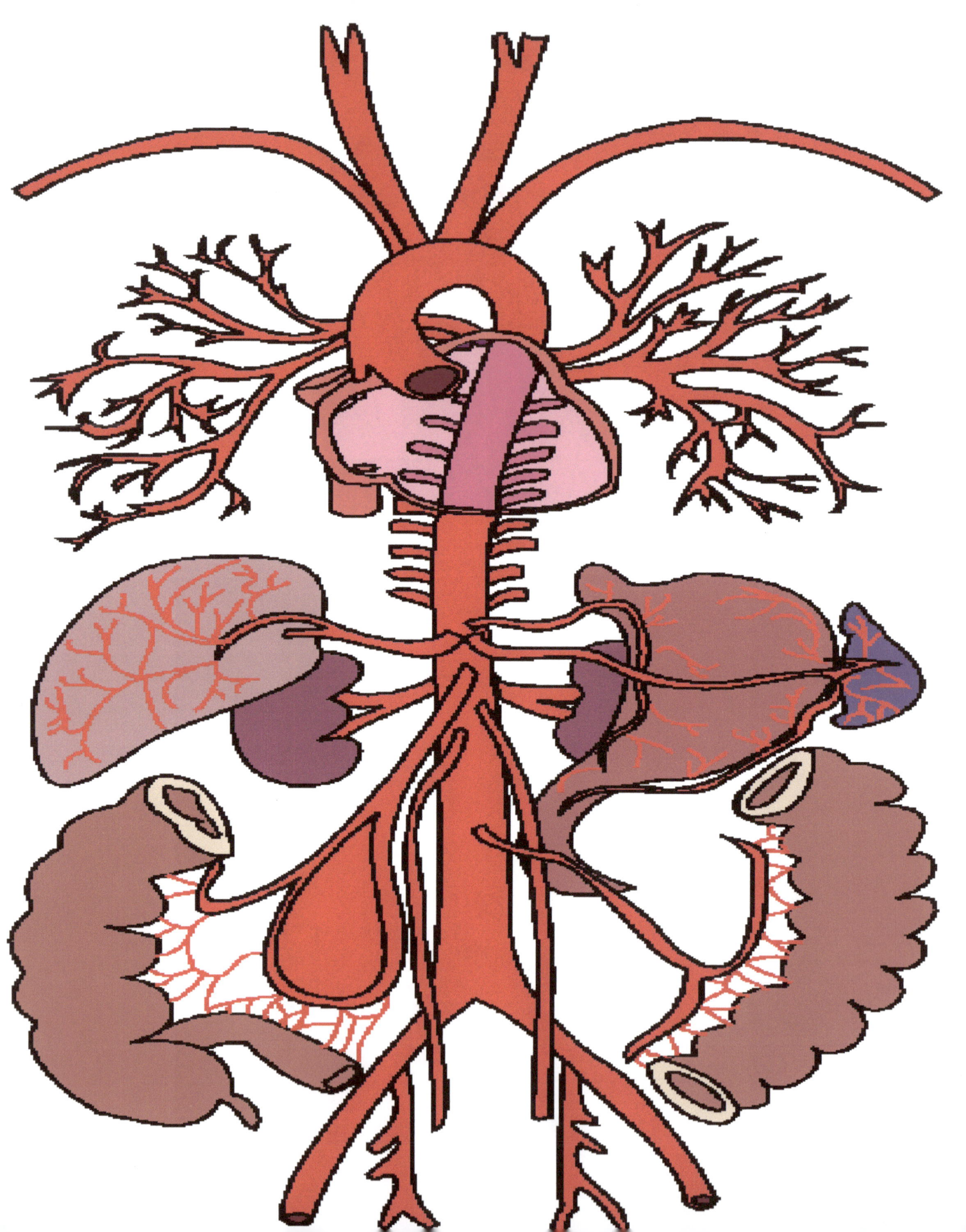

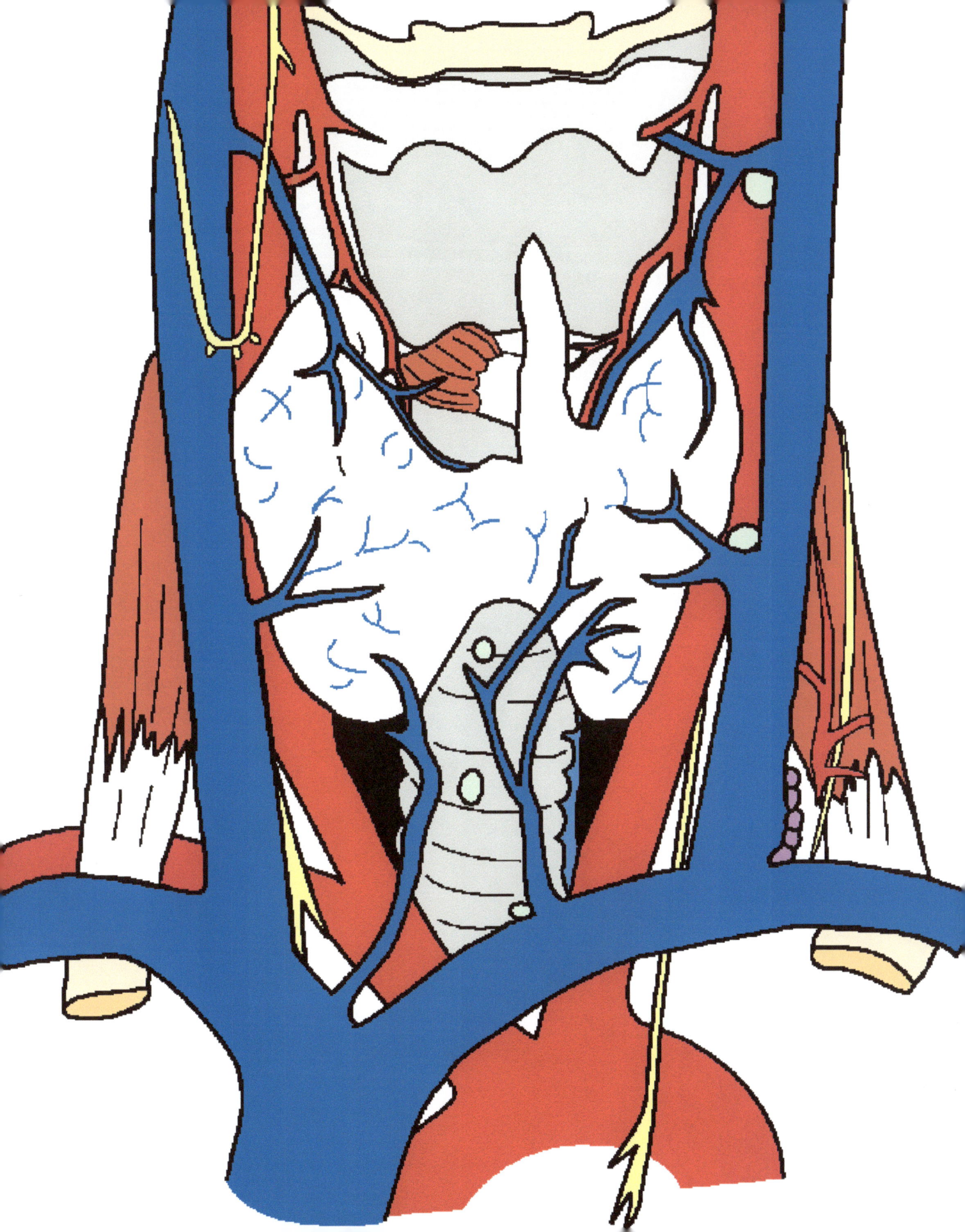

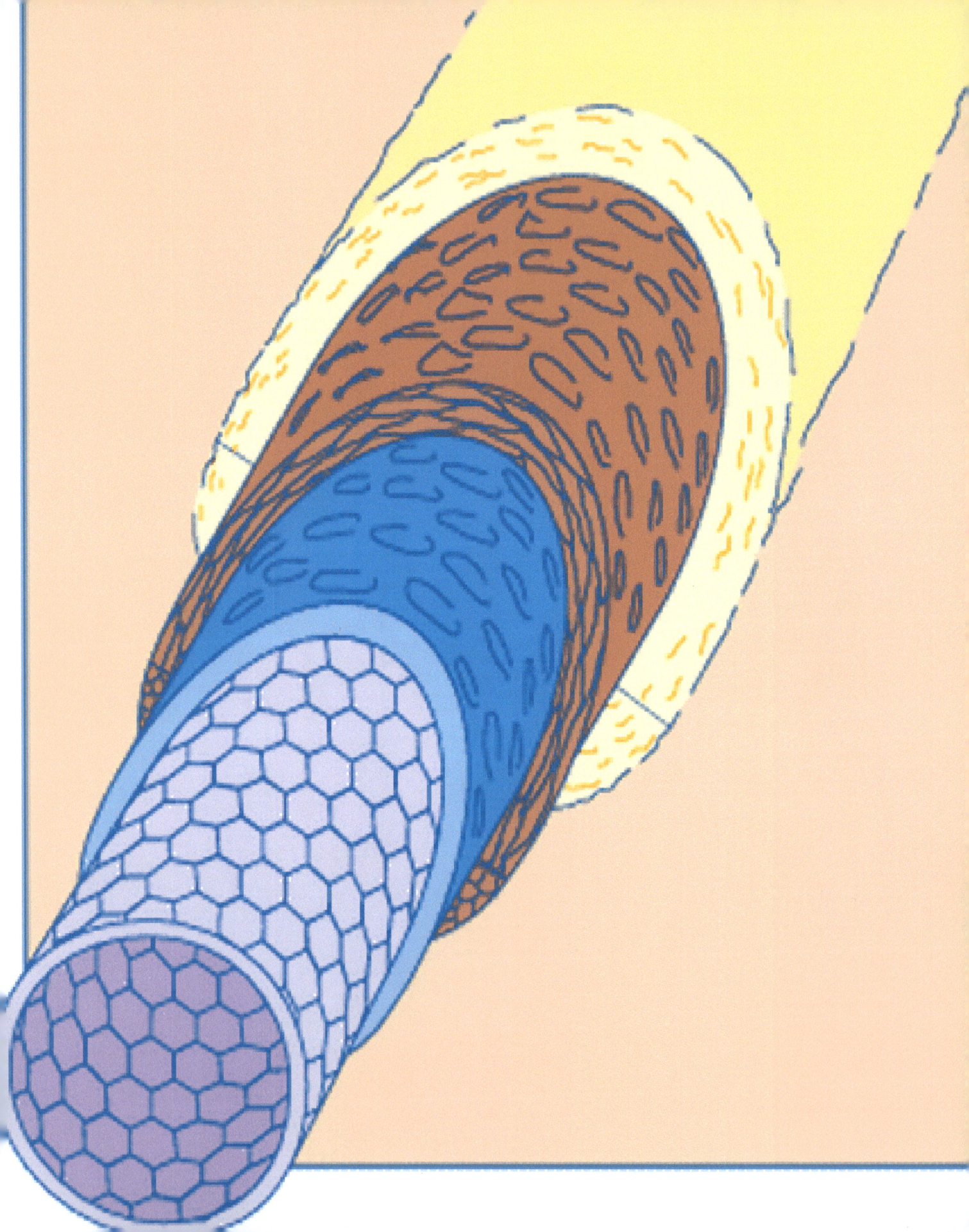

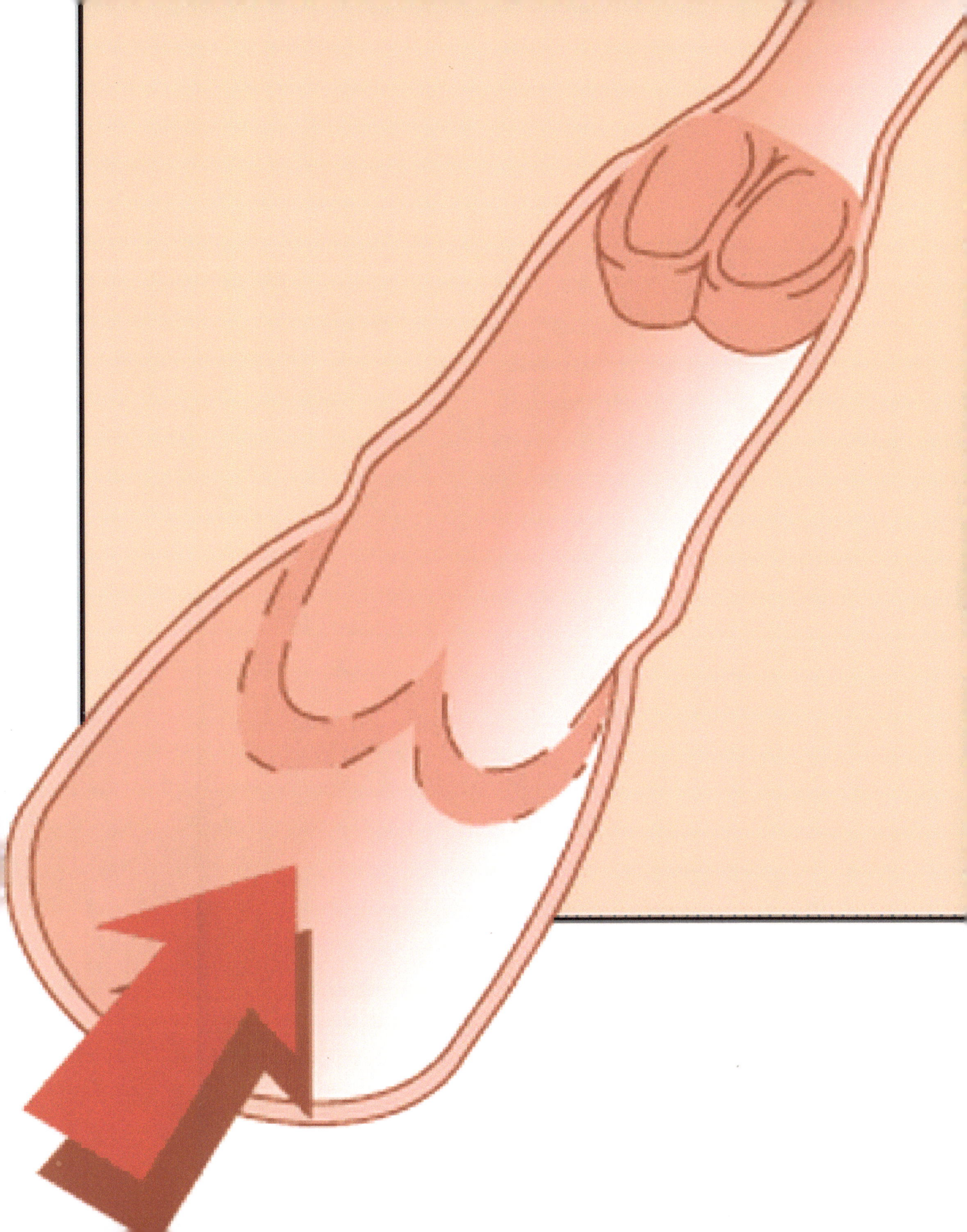

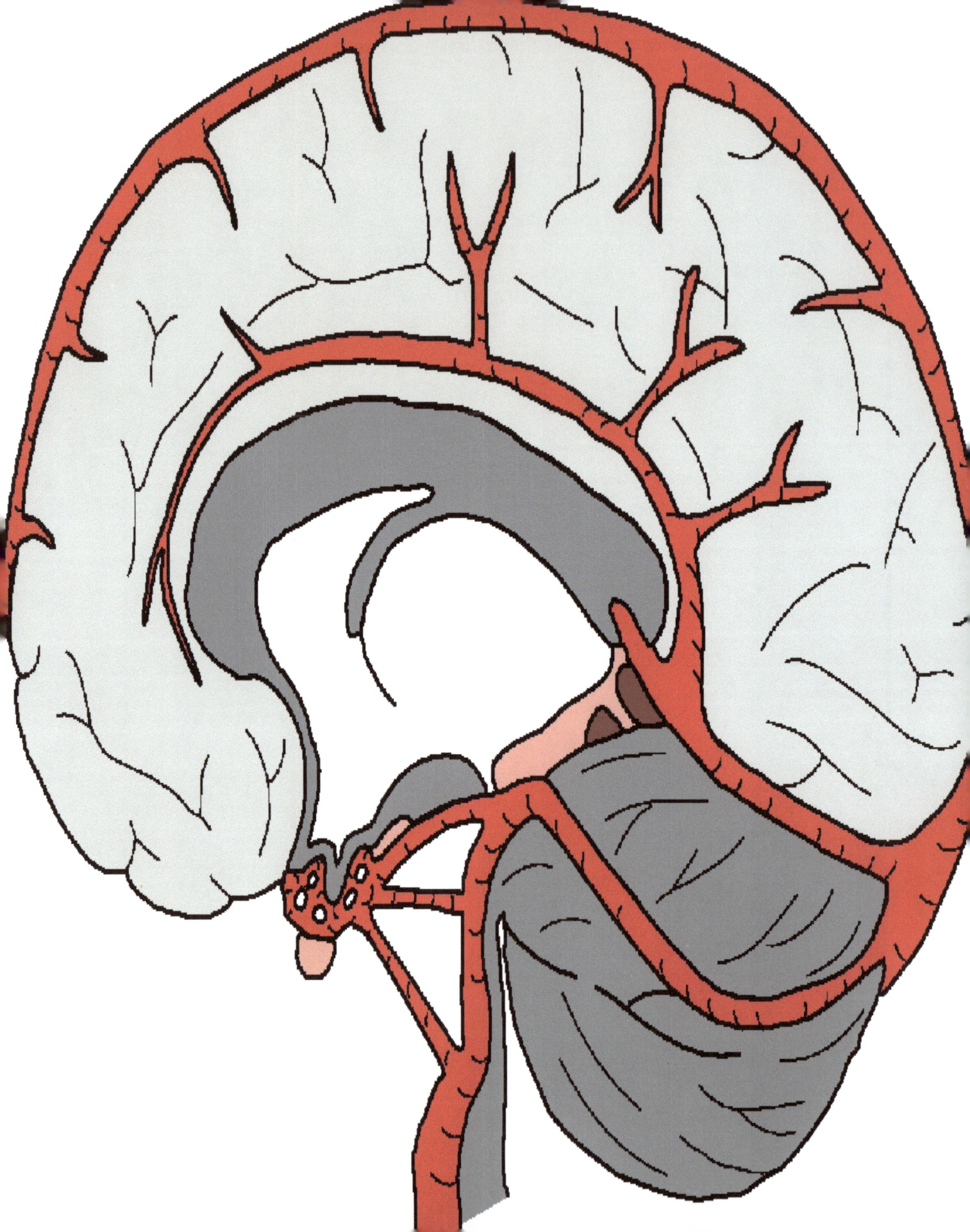

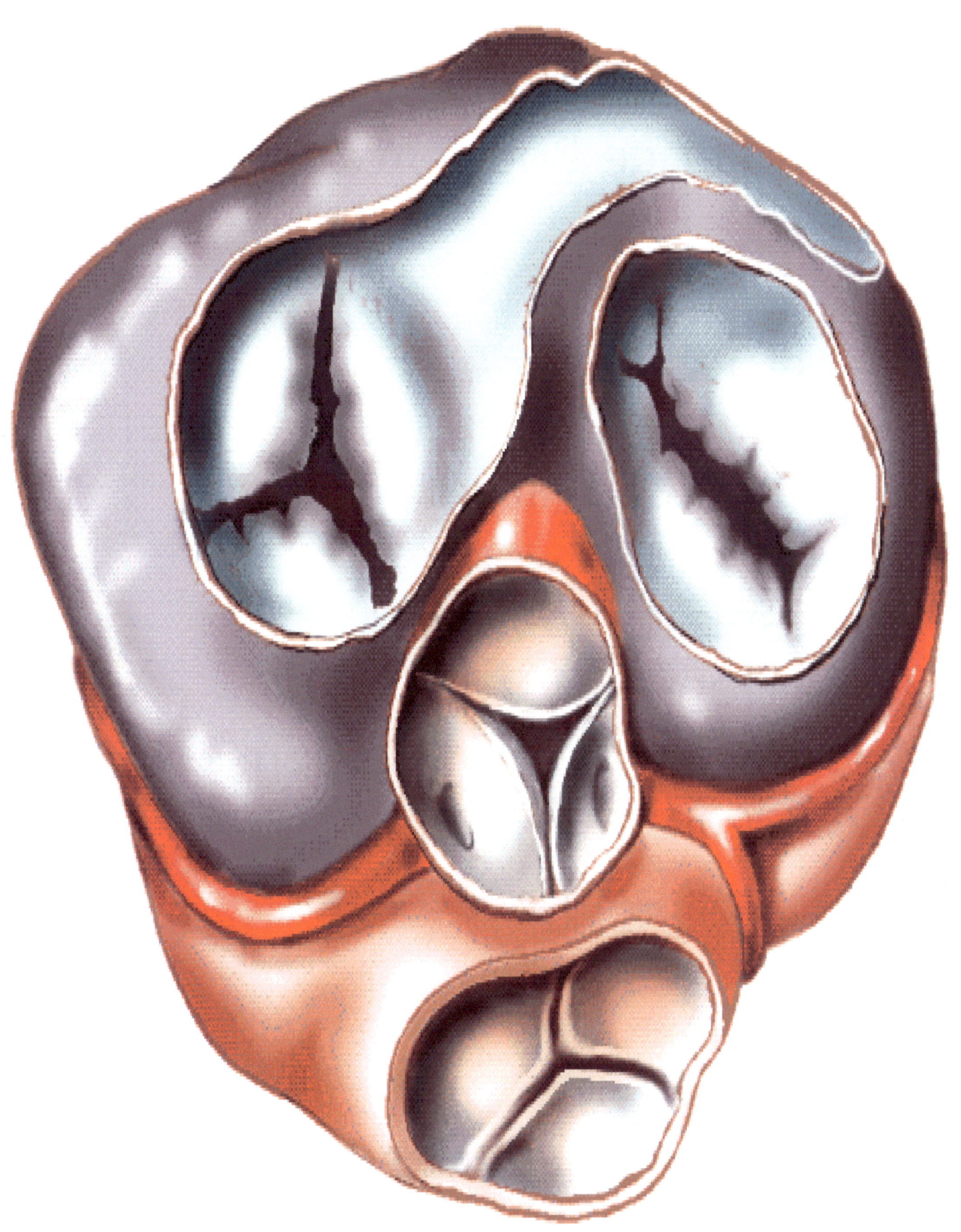

Other Anatomy System Label Practice <u>Books Available on</u> <u>Amazon</u>

1. Cardiovascular System
2. Digestive & Endocrine System
3. Muscular System
4. Nervous System
5. Respiratory System
6. Skeleteal System
7. Surface Anatomy & Senses
8. Urogenital System

www.ingramcontent.com/pod-product-compliance
Lightning Source LLC
Chambersburg PA
CBHW050729180526
45159CB00003B/1173